LEE RODWELL is an experienced journalist, with a special interest in health matters. In Britain she writes for several national newspapers – including *The Times* and *Independent* – as well as a variety of magazines. Her articles have also appeared in publications around the world.

She is the author of two reference books for women. Married, with two children, she lives in North London.

Women
and
Medical Care

Women
and
Medical Care

Lee Rodwell

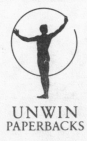

UNWIN
PAPERBACKS

LONDON SYDNEY WELLINGTON

First published in Great Britain by Unwin® Paperbacks, an imprint of Unwin
Hyman Limited in 1988

UNWIN HYMAN LIMITED
15/17 Broadwick Street, London W1V 1FP

Allen & Unwin Australia Pty Ltd
8 Napier Street, North Sydney, NSW 2060, Australia

Allen & Unwin New Zealand Pty Ltd with Port Nicholson Press
60 Cambridge Terrace, Wellington, New Zealand

British Library Cataloguing in Publication Data
Rodwell, Lee
    Everywoman guide to women and health.
1. Women. Health – For women
I. Title
613′.04244

ISBN 0–04–440293–7

Set in 11 on 12 point Ehrhardt by Computape (Pickering) Ltd, North Yorkshire
and printed in Great Britain by The Guernsey Press Co. Ltd,
Guernsey, Channel Islands.

CONTENTS

INTRODUCTION:
WOMEN AND MEDICAL CARE

At some point in our lives we all need medical care, whether it is treatment for a minor infection or major surgery. Often women have particular needs relating to their sex, from advice on how to find the right kind of contraception, to help in overcoming difficulties created by the menopause.

However, getting the right kind of medical care is not always as easy as it might be. Even finding out what is available can be a difficult task, as the provision of services varies from place to place and from time to time, and, in any case, is not always widely publicised.

In addition, women are often reluctant to 'make a fuss' or 'take up the doctor's time', although they would not hesitate to take their children to the doctor's surgery, and willingly spend time and trouble supporting their husbands and other members of their families when they are ill.

Sometimes, too, when women do eventually seek help, they encounter attitudes that may be discouraging. There are still doctors, for instance, who are unsympathetic about requests for help with premenstrual tension or painful episiotomy scars.

This book aims to give women the information they need to make the most of the services that are available, both within the National Health Service and outside it, in the private sector.

It is not meant to be a campaigning book – although, goodness knows, there are enough topics one could campaign about – nor is it a defence of, or an attack upon, the National Health Service. During the period I was writing and researching this book, the problems facing the health service were much in the news. I doubt whether, by the time you read this, they will all have been solved and that is all the more reason why I hope you will find it useful.

In the first part of the book I have tried to outline the way the health services are set up. Then I have dealt with the people you are most likely to meet and the type of care they offer. Finally, I have turned to the individual problems you might have, tackling each subject in alphabetical order.

Knowing how the system works and what kind of support is available is part of the equation. But feeling confident enough to make use of that knowledge is another. After all, when we become patients we also become consumers, yet many of us feel far less sure of ourselves than we do in other areas of our lives. Shopping around for a fridge-freezer that will suit our needs is one thing; shopping around for a GP who will do the same feels entirely different. In the final analysis, however, the latter is really more important.

So how can we gain the confidence we need? In recent years the concept of assertiveness has become very popular and many books and courses have been devoted to the subject. Some of the techniques suggested can be used quite success-fully in doctor/patient situations.

To begin with, you have to recognise the difference between assertion and aggression – losing your temper, shouting, refusing to listen, being rude; all these aggressive patterns of behaviour are unhelpful. But you do not have to go to the other extreme, passively accepting whatever is done to you.

Being assertive means taking responsibility for your own actions, making your own choices, feeling able to voice your own needs and, if necessary, negotiate a satisfactory solution.

The trouble is that it can be difficult to feel assertive when we are dealing with someone who appears to have more status or power than we do, and doctors and nurses often fall into this category. They wear white coats, or uniforms, or sit behind desks. They are the ones who look in control.

Some women say it helps to imagine these 'authority figures' in ludicrous situations. 'I had a particularly pompous consultant, who saw me during my pregnancy,' said a friend of mine, 'and in order to summon up the nerve to speak to the "Big Chief" I used to think about him sitting in the bath with no clothes on.'

Frivolous? Maybe. But worth a try if it will help. It should also help to remind yourself that although this consultant or that GP has more specific expert knowledge than you, that knowledge is there for your benefit, and you still have the right to be treated as an equal human being.

One way of getting this equal treatment is to plan ahead. Before your appointment, think about what you are going to say. To start with, you can work out the answers to the questions you are likely to be asked. You are bound to be asked about your symptoms, when they started, whether they have been getting worse, what effect they are having on your daily life. You will probably be asked if you have taken any

2

medicines and, if so, what effect they had. You might be asked the date of your last period, or other questions about the regularity of your menstrual cycle or gynaecological history. You might be asked about any related problems you, or anyone else in your family (your sister, your mother) have had in the past.

Think about what you are going to wear, too. If there is a chance you will be examined, choose something that makes it easy for you to dress and undress. If you are going to have your blood pressure checked, you will need sleeves that can be rolled up.

The next step is to sort out what it is you want from the doctor and how to ask for it. There are a number of techniques which may be useful. First of all you should be specific:

- I want to stop smoking and I'd like your help.
- I'm still suffering from PMS (premenstrual syndrome) and I'd like to be referred to a specialist.
- My pregnancy test is positive and I'd like to talk about the alternatives for antenatal care and delivery.
- I'm feeling dreadful and I want to know what's the matter with me.

It is actually quite difficult to come right out and say what you want. Most of us beat around the bush a bit, throwing in phrases like, 'I'm sorry to be such a nuisance, but I wondered if it might be possible . . .'. You might need to practise at home first.

Another technique you will probably need to practise is that of sticking to your guns. Get someone else to play the role of the difficult doctor – or play that role yourself and see how your counterpart handles the situation.

Try to work out ways of fielding all possible responses and restating your request without getting sidetracked.

- I know willpower is important, but I'd still like your help.
- I appreciate that PMS is very common, but I'd still like to see a specialist.
- I understand that most women go to the local maternity unit, but I'd still like to talk about the other possibilities too.

Often what we want from doctors is more information. As patients, we have no right of access to our medical records and sometimes – unless we ask directly – we will not actually be told what is wrong with us. Even when we are told, we may not fully understand, or we may come out of the surgery with the

3

feeling that everything went in one ear and straight out of the other.

In her book, *A Woman In Your Own Right*, Anne Dickson says we should all remind ourselves that we have a basic human right to say we do not understand. 'With this right in mind you can learn to acknowledge confusion or non-comprehension without feeling stupid. You can learn to ask for more information or a repeated explanation without feeling ridiculous.'

Another tip which may help to fix the information in your mind is to repeat what you have been told, in your own words. 'So what you are saying, doctor, is . . .' That way you will know you have got it right.

Getting what you want is one side of the coin; not having to accept treatment that you do not want is the other. Although there are a few exceptions (related to mental patients or notifiable infectious diseases), your consent is needed before any medical treatment can be carried out. (In an emergency, if a patient is unconscious, a doctor can carry out treatment to save life, but any treatment which could wait must do so until the patient can give his or her informed consent.)

Consent can either be implied (in other words, your behaviour made it clear that you accepted the course of treatment), or express (you sign an operation consent form, for example). Of course, you do not have to give your consent until you are sure in your own mind about everything involved. And if you are not really sure, ask for time to think about it, and also ask for any extra information you need to help you to make your decision.

Self-help can play a part in this. To make the most of the medical care that is available, and to fill the gaps where it is not, it is often necessary to find out as much as we can ourselves about a particular problem.

The idea that we can assume control of our own health, and take steps to improve the way we live and the way we feel, has become increasingly popular, and there is a growing number of self-help groups and organisations which can give you the information and support to do this.

Even when you are getting all the medical care possible, a self-help group can help you to understand what is going on and can provide the kind of back-up that makes a positive difference.

Throughout this book, where relevant, I have included

details of groups of this kind. All the addresses and telephone numbers are listed on pages 93–97 and are as up to date as I could make them, but please do not lose heart if some of them have changed. If you have problems tracking down a particular organisation, try your Community Health Council or local library.

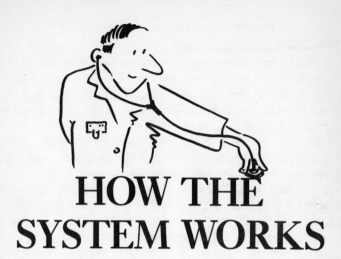

HOW THE
SYSTEM WORKS

THE NATIONAL HEALTH SERVICE

The primary health care services

The primary health care services can be seen as the front line of the NHS and they carry an enormous workload. Each year, for instance, there are some 190 million consultations with family doctors in England and Wales – yet only a minority of the people who are seen (around 10 per cent) are referred to hospital or specialist services.

The primary health care services fulfil three main roles: diagnosing and treating illness; preventing illness; and providing comfort and support for the community.

In England and Wales some of the primary health care services are ultimately the responsibility of Family Practitioner Committees. These are the services provided outside hospital by family doctors, dentists, pharmacists and opticians.

Others, such as the services provided by community nurses, midwives, health visitors and other professions allied to medicine, are the responsibility of Regional and District Health Authorities.

The kind of things provided by these community health services vary from area to area, but they would, for instance, be responsible for running a variety of clinics, from family planning to child development, cervical cytology (smear tests) to chiropody, physiotherapy to parentcraft. They are also responsible for running the school health programmes.

The set-up is slightly different in Scotland and Northern Ireland. In Scotland there are Health Boards, each with its own Primary Care Division which arranges contracts with GPs, dentists, pharmacists and opticians. In Northern Ireland these contracts are held by the Health and Social Service Boards through the Central Services Agency.

Secondary health care

If you have a medical problem which is an emergency, or needs further investigation or surgery, then the chances are that you will need to go to a hospital. If it is an emergency, you will probably be sent straight to an Accident and Emergency Unit. Otherwise your GP will write a letter, referring you to the relevant out-patient clinic, and you will be contacted by them and given a date for an appointment to see a specialist, usually a consultant. If it proves necessary for you to be admitted to hospital, the specialist will so refer you, and on admission you will become an in-patient.

Some hospitals run clinics for women with premenstrual or menopausal problems. However, provision often depends on funding and the interests of a particular consultant, and where such clinics exist, demand often exceeds supply.

Hospitals also provide specialist services, such as physiotherapy and occupational therapy.

THE PRIVATE SECTOR

The vast majority of people still rely on the NHS for their primary health care, although there are some GPs who take private patients. (There are more of these in London than elsewhere.)

However, about five and a half million people now belong to health insurance schemes and prefer to go outside the NHS if they need to see a specialist. The private sector is capable of treating patients with all kinds of conditions, from relatively minor complaints to all acute medical and surgical cases, including cardiac surgery and transplants, and there are just over 200 private hospitals, and around 3,000 pay-beds, in NHS hospitals.

In certain circumstances, private health insurance may not fully cover you – if, for instance, it turns out that you are suffering from a longterm incurable condition. In addition, pregnancy and childbirth are seen as normal conditions, so, unless there are complications, you would have to foot this bill yourself if you wanted to be seen privately. (See page 69.)

FINDING OUT WHAT'S AVAILABLE

There are a number of ways of finding out what medical services are available in your area, and in 1987 the government announced new measures to help people to do this.

They said they were going to talk to the General Medical Council about allowing doctors to advertise (subject to proper safeguards), which was previously forbidden. They also said they were going to encourage more family doctors to produce leaflets about themselves and their services. In fact, some practices already do this.

Of course, once you have registered with a GP, he or she should be able to tell you all about the local services on offer, including the consultants who take private patients and whether there are any independent hospitals or clinics.

Community Health Councils

Another useful source of information, if you live in England or Wales, can be your local Community Health Council. You will find the address in the local telephone directory, or you can contact the Association of Community Health Councils of England and Wales (ACHEW). In Scotland the equivalent of the CHCs are the Local Health Councils; in Northern Ireland they are called District Committees.

Community Health Councils were set up to act as independent local voices on health matters, to represent the interests of people living, working or using the services in their area. This is a good place to start if you are trying to find out about either NHS primary care or hospital services. Your CHC can help with individual queries, problems or complaints, either directly or by putting you in touch with another agency.

Many CHCs also produce a number of useful publications. Ealing Community Health Council, for instance, has compiled a comprehensive *Good Health Guide* which is a mine of information about local health-related services. Another London Community Health Council, Barnet, has its own *Woman's Guide to Health in Barnet*.

The Family Practitioner Committee

The Family Practitioner Committee provides lists of GPs, which can generally be found at main post offices, town halls, libraries and the local Community Health Council office. In 1987, the government said it intended to require FPCs and health boards to provide more comprehensive information about practices in their area.

Future lists, said the government, should include not only names and addresses of GPs, but also each doctor's year of qualification, sex and qualifications, as well as essential practice information, such as surgery hours, services provided, and arrangements for emergency and night calls.

Other organisations which may provide information, support or help include:

Women's Health Concern

A registered charity, set up in 1980, WHC answers some 20,000 enquiries each year from women all over Britain, mainly about gynaecological problems, treatment and preventative care. It provides a specialist advisory service for menopause and PMS sufferers and can arrange counselling sessions, for a fee. It also publishes books and booklets on a variety of subjects. All letters must include an s.a.e. (See page 97.)

Women's Health Information Centre

This is a national information and resource centre for women's health issues. (See page 96.)

The Patients' Association

This is an independent organisation which gives advice on using the NHS, sorting out difficulties and making complaints. Publications include *Using the NHS*; *Can I Insist?*; *Advice on Going into Hospital*; *A Guide to Patients' Legal Rights*. The association also produces a self-help directory at £2.95. Membership is £5 per annum, but you do not have to be a member to seek advice by telephoning on either Tuesday or Thursday during office hours. (See page 95.)

The Medical Advisory Service

This is a charity which can offer help and advice on most medical topics, although the nurses who run it cannot diagnose or recommend particular doctors or hospitals. However, they can explain what you are entitled to, and how to go about getting it. If they feel you would benefit by contacting someone else, they will pass you on to the right body. (See page 94.)

The reference section of your local library is often a good source of information. For instance, it may have a copy of the *Hospitals and Health Services Year Book*. You can use this to find out which hospitals serve your area, and whether or not those hospitals have any private beds.

Another book well worth getting hold of is *A Patient's Guide to the National Health Service*.

For the private sector, you may find the *Directory of Independent Hospitals and Health Services* useful. Once you have identified your local private hospitals, you can ring up the director of each and ask which specialists use the hospital.

11

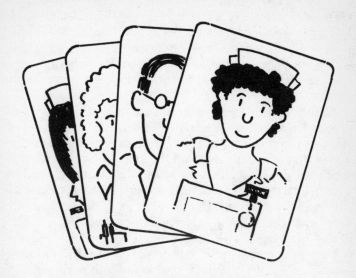

THE PEOPLE

GENERAL PRACTITIONERS

GPs (family doctors), working in the NHS, are employed by Family Practitioner Committees as independent contractors to provide general medical services for people who register with them. They are paid according to the number of people on their list, plus extra payments for certain additional items.

At the time of writing, the government is proposing the biggest shake-up of GP services since 1948. The idea is to relate pay to performance, by changing the existing structure and setting up a new one, with the emphasis on preventative medicine, in which doctors would be paid for reaching specified targets for breast and cervical screening, vaccination and immunisation programmes. Doctors would be paid extra for regular checks on the elderly and for specialising in child health.

Under the new scheme, GPs would also be given financial incentives to carry out minor operations in their surgeries, to ease hospital workloads, and they would be forced to retire at seventy.

Whether all, or some, or none of this has come to pass by the time you read this book, your GP will still be your first port of call under most circumstances, so finding a doctor with whom you can have a good relationship is vital. However, that is not always easy. Even registering with a doctor can be difficult in some parts of the country.

Finding a GP

On your medical card you will find the address of the Family Practitioner Committee, who publish a complete list of NHS doctors in your area and their surgery times. Alternatively, you may find this list at your local library, Citizen's Advice Bureau or post office. The local Community Health Council will also have one.

If you have lost your medical card, you can contact the Society of Family Practitioner Committees and they will tell you how to get a new one. You will find the address and telephone number of your Family Practitioner Committee in your local telephone directory.

At present, the list itself gives the minimum information about the range of services each practice offers. It might state the surgery hours and tell you what kind of appointment system applies. You ought to be able to see whether doctors are male or female and when they first registered. The list should also tell you if a particular doctor provides family planning services and whether or not this service applies to anyone, or only patients registered with that doctor. It will also indicate which GPs are qualified to care for women during pregnancy and childbirth.

However, the extent of the care offered to pregnant women varies. While many GPs provide antenatal care (usually on a shared-care basis with a hospital), relatively few will actually attend the delivery of your baby, either at a GP unit at a local hospital, or at home. (See page 65.)

This is the kind of information you will not be able to get from the list, nor will it tell you what particular interests each doctor has (whether he or she uses acupuncture, or other forms of alternative medicine; if there is a special clinic for asthmatic or diabetic patients, or for smokers who want to stop), and it certainly will not be able to tell you whether one GP is particularly involved in the problems of the elderly, while another takes a special interest in children.

Some practices have a nurse – either a district nurse, who comes to the surgery, or a nurse employed directly by the practice. Depending on their training and qualifications, these nurses may carry out a variety of tasks from ear syringing and changing dressings, to administering routine childhood vaccinations, carrying out breast examinations and cervical smears, or other health checks, such as testing for sugar in urine (a sign of diabetes), or high blood pressure.

So how can you find out exactly what each surgery offers? The government wants to make it easier for people to choose the right GP for them. To this end, they want more information to be included on the medical lists; they want more practices to produce practice leaflets; and they want the General Medical Council to lift the restraint on doctors advertising their services.

All this will help, but the time-honoured way of finding out about GPs is to ask your friends and neighbours for their opinions, and this still holds good. It is also worth visiting any surgery you are considering, to speak with the staff there. You should not feel guilty about wasting their valuable time, says Mrs Gallagher of the Society of Family Practitioners: 'Unless there is a good doctor/patient relationship, you are not going to get very far.'

The *Medical Register*, which you might find in the reference section of your library, lists all doctors in the area and will tell you when a doctor qualified, so you may be able to get some idea of his or her age. It lists qualifications, research interests and papers published, so it can also give you an idea of a doctor's special interests. Also available is the *Medical Directory* which lists some but not all doctors.

Another point to consider is whether it is worth going to a practice based at a health centre. Often two or three different surgeries are based at one health centre, and under these circumstances the practices may club together to buy and share various items of equipment. This may mean they are better equipped than smaller individual practices elsewhere, and, in general, the facilities may be of a high standard. On the other hand, a large group practice outside a health centre may be similarly equipped in any case.

It is also a good idea to establish exactly what kind of appointment system the various practices have. Will it be easy to see a doctor in a hurry? What is the policy on home visits? Are the surgery hours convenient for you? Will you normally be able to see the same GP each time? What arrangements are made for cover at night or weekends? How helpful does the receptionist appear to be?

You should also bear in mind that GPs, like everyone else, are entitled to time off. This means that in an emergency – particularly at weekends and during the night – you may find yourself dealing with a deputising service.

Can I insist on a woman doctor?

Many women prefer to be seen by a woman GP – but no one can insist on this. Even if you eventually register with a woman doctor, if she works with men in a group practice you may have to resign yourself to being seen by her colleagues from time to time, unless you are always prepared to wait for an appointment with her. On occasions, this could be a matter of weeks rather than days.

Obviously, if there are two or three women working in a group practice, the odds of seeing a woman doctor every time are much higher.

Closed lists

Once you have done your homework, you will have to find out whether or not the doctor of your choice will accept you. Some practices feel that they already have enough patients to cope with adequately and so their lists are closed.

Unless you live in a rural area, you may find that GPs only accept new patients who live quite near to their surgeries. This has to do with home visits – obviously a doctor can fit in more home visits if the patients live nearby, than if they are scattered over a wider area.

The upshot of this is that all your investigations can go by the board and you may find yourself left with no real choice at all. You may even despair of getting on *anyone's* list.

You have a right to GP care, however, and, under these circumstances, you should write to the Family Practitioner Committee, who will assign you to a doctor who will be instructed to take you onto his or her list.

How to register

In most cases, you simply fill in Part A on your medical card and hand this in to your new doctor. He or she signs the card and sends it on to the FPC for registration.

The FPC will then send you a new card. You do not have to be registered with the same GP as your husband, your parents or your children, although it may be sensible if everyone in the same family has the same doctor. Under-sixteens have to be registered by their parents.

Changing doctors

Most of us only change doctors when we move house. But sometimes people want to change because they are unhappy with the relationship they have with their GP, or for some other reason. If such is the case, there are at present two ways of going about this, although, as part of the shake-up of GP services, the government is proposing to make the process simpler by changing the regulations so that you can register directly with a new doctor without going through either of the procedures outlined below.

● Ask your present doctor for his or her consent to you transferring to the doctor of your choice. You can do this by writing a letter, if you do not want to meet your present doctor face to face. If the doctor agrees, you ask him or her to sign Part B of your medical card and then you and your new doctor complete Part A in the usual way.

● If, however, you do not want to ask your doctor directly for his or her consent – or if he or she refuses to give it –

you can send your medical card direct to the FPC with a letter explaining that you wish to transfer to Dr X. You do not have to give a reason, although you can do so if you wish.

The FPA will return your medical card, along with a slip giving you permission to transfer after a stated date. The slip is valid for a month, so if you still want to go ahead, you must do so within this time.

You complete Part 1 of the transfer slip and take or send it, with your medical card, to the new doctor. If the new doctor accepts you, he or she signs Part 2 of the slip and you are then on that doctor's list. You will be sent a new medical card later.

Sometimes doctors refuse to take patients from another doctor's list if they are both based in the same area. While this means you may not have much choice as to who your new doctor will be, it does not mean you have to stay with your old doctor.

If you cannot find a new doctor yourself, then write to the FPC, telling them the name or names of doctors who have refused you and of any doctors with whom you would prefer not to be registered. They will assign you to a suitable doctor.

Emergencies

If you are away from home and need a doctor in an emergency – or if your own doctor is not available for some reason – you are entitled to treatment on the NHS from any local doctor. If you are away from home for less than three months, you can apply to a doctor for acceptance as a temporary patient. If you are living away from home for more than three months you should register with a local doctor.

Private GP care

Some GPs treat patients privately (and the present Conservative Government sees no reason why more should not do so). The only way to find out if particular doctors take private patients is to contact them and ask.

Fees will vary, but the average consultation will probably cost between £30 and £35. You will have to pay any prescription charges on top of this.

Many doctors – even those who take private patients – argue that there is little to be gained by seeing a GP privately.

One told me: 'My appointments book is full for the next

three weeks, so you are hardly cutting out the waiting time. And in any case, if it was an emergency your NHS GP would see you straightaway. Probably the only advantages are that you would be more likely to get a home visit and you might get half an hour of the doctor's time at each appointment, rather than ten minutes.'

GP services you have to pay for

There are some services, provided by your GP, which you will have to pay for. If you need innoculations before you go abroad on business or on a holiday, for instance, or if you require a private medical certificate, or to have a private health insurance form signed, your GP can charge.

Making complaints

If you have a complaint to make about the standard of service provided by your GP – and you feel you have got nowhere by discussing the matter directly with the doctor or doctors involved – you can write to the Family Practitioner Committee (see page 14). You must do this within eight weeks of the incident about which you are complaining. Your local Community Health Council should be able to help you if you need advice or if you feel your complaint has not been satisfactorily dealt with.

In the past, many people have criticised the way the complaints system works and, as a result, the government is proposing to simplify and streamline procedures. This would mean, amongst other things, that you could complain verbally, rather than in writing, and the time limit would be extended from eight to thirteen weeks.

Complaints about a GP's behaviour, professional responsibility, or ethical conduct should be made to the General Medical Council. (See page 95.)

Getting a second opinion

In most cases your GP will automatically refer you to a specialist if he or she thinks your particular problem warrants it. However, there are times when you may be unhappy about the way a GP is dealing with you, and you yourself would prefer a second opinion. In cases like this, you should ask to be referred for one. If you are covered by private health insurance, you should point this out, and if you wish to be referred to a particular specialist, you should make this clear too.

Most GPs are reasonably happy about referring patients who ask for a second opinion from a specialist, either to confirm their own diagnosis, or to get difficult people off their backs. However, while you are entitled to ask for a second opinion, your GP is not obliged to refer you for one. He or she may suggest that you see one of the other GPs if it is a group practice, but if you want to see a specialist and your request is flatly refused, your only recourse is to complain to your FPC, or to change GPs.

Incidentally, if you are going to see a specialist and expect the bills to be met through an insurance scheme, do not be afraid to ask what the specialist's fee will be. Health insurance schemes have fixed limits on certain fees and, although most doctors who take private patients know what the structure is, you should make sure you are covered.

Also, if you are going to be admitted to hospital, check that it is not outside your banding, or else you will have to pay the extra amount.

COMMUNITY NURSES

There are around 50,000 nurses who work outside hopsitals. Some become health visitors or district nurses, others work in places like family planning clinics or in the school health programmes, and some are employed by GPs as practice nurses. Some also work as community midwives.

District nurses

District, or home nurses take care of people who have been discharged from hospital and still need nursing. They also visit people at home, who need particular drugs administered regularly, or who need injections or to have dressings changed. If you need the services of a district nurse, then you should be referred by your GP or a hospital-based consultant.

School nurses

School nurses are employed by the education authority and their work involves keeping an eye on children's health. They will check on immunization and whether or not children have had booster jabs, and they also keep an eye out for things like head lice.

Practice nurses

Practice nurses are employed by some GPs. Different practices offer different services. Some practices give a nurse her own treatment room where she may carry out a variety of tasks, from syringing ears to giving vaccinations, or run screening tests, such as blood pressure and urine checks. Ask your GP what services are available.

Health visitors

Health visitors are nurses who have had a year's special training on how to teach people about healthy living. They visit people at home and also give advice in clinics. Health visitors contact mums-to-be to offer support and advice and then keep in touch once the baby is born. They also run baby and child health clinics. Health visitors can give advice about diet, smoking and accident prevention, and have a particular interest in the needs of the young, the elderly and the disabled. They can also give advice and information about what the health and social services have to offer. You can contact a health visitor through your local child care clinic.

Community midwives

Community midwives are often involved in antenatal care and are responsible for Domino and home deliveries (see page 68). They usually make a point of getting to know mothers-to-be before they have their babies (wherever this is going to happen) and they also visit new mothers at home from the time they leave hospital until ten days after the birth, during which time they check on the progress of both mother and baby.

SPECIALISTS AND CONSULTANTS

If your GP thinks you need to see a specialist, he or she will usually decide which one to refer you to. If you have any particular preferences, you should discuss these with the GP. You might also prefer to go to one hospital rather than another, so discuss this possibility too. This applies whether you are going to be treated under the NHS or privately.

Unless you are going in as a private patient, you cannot insist on seeing the consultant and may, in fact, be dealt with by his or her registrar or house officer.

Waiting lists (out-patients)

How long you will have to wait to see a specialist depends on a number of factors including the urgency of your particular case, what is wrong with you, which consultant you are due to see, and where you live. Waiting lists for different kinds of specialities vary up and down the country. Your GP should know what local conditions are like, so ask when the referral is made. You may prefer to travel some distance if it means you will be seen sooner – your GP does not automatically have to refer you to the nearest hospital.

If you can afford it, or if you are covered by private health insurance, you can cut the waiting time by seeing a consultant privately. After this initial consultation, you can always revert to the NHS for any in-patient treatment, although you could not insist that the same consultant carried this out.

Waiting lists (in-patients)

The waiting times for admission to hospital vary. If you think you have been waiting too long, you could ask your GP to contact the hospital again to see what is happening. You could also ask the Admissions Department, or the sister in charge of the out-patients clinic you attended, whether the hospital keeps a list of patients who can come in at short notice (this may be a matter of hours).

Second opinions

After you have seen a specialist as an out-patient, your GP should receive a letter outlining the proposed treatment of your case. You do not have to accept any treatment suggested, and if you have any doubts, your GP should be able to help you to decide. Your GP will also be able to explain anything you did not understand at the time of your consultation. If you are still not happy, you can ask to be referred to another consultant.

Complaints

If you have a complaint about the treatment you have had or are getting, or about a doctor's clinical judgement, you should contact the consultant concerned. If this gets you nowhere, you should write to the hospital administrator, if you have been dealt with under the NHS. If you are a private patient, then your consultant's care is a matter of private contract between the two of you. If your complaint is about the personal, ethical or professional behaviour of a doctor, then you should write to the General Medical Council (see page 95).

Complaints about other hospital employees or services should be made to the hospital administrator or the district administrator. If you need advice, ask your local Community Health Council.

Negligence

Everyone has the right in law to be treated with reasonable care and reasonable skill. But sometimes things go badly wrong, and if a patient suffers as a result of professional negligence, then she is entitled to sue for compensation or damages. This holds good whether you are a private or an NHS patient.

However, proving that a doctor failed to provide reasonable skill or care is not always easy, and you would need supporting medical opinion and legal advice.

If you are considering suing (and this is often a lengthy and expensive business) you would be well advised to seek help initially from a local neighbourhood law centre, if there is one, or a Citizen's Advice Bureau. It may also be possible to find a solicitor who operates the fixed-fee scheme, whereby you pay a fixed fee for a fixed-time interview to explore the possibilities of legal action. To find out if any local solicitors operate this scheme, you would have to look up 'Solicitors' in the Yellow Pages and ring around.

WOMEN'S HEALTH FROM

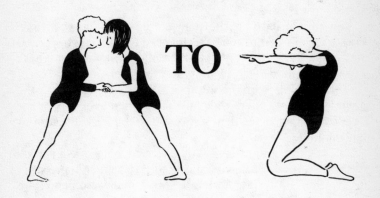

TO

ABORTION

If you are pregnant and do not want to have the baby, then you should act quickly. At the time of writing, abortion is legal up to twenty-eight weeks of pregnancy, but there have been campaigns to reduce this legal limit to eighteen weeks. In any event, for practical reasons, few abortions are carried out later than twenty-four weeks, and the earlier this is done, the easier and safer it is.

You cannot have an abortion just because you want one. Under the 1967 Abortion Act, you need two doctors to agree – and sign a form to that effect – that in their opinion you have sufficient grounds. These are either that there is a real risk of the baby being born handicapped, or that continuing the pregnancy would affect your physical or mental health, or the physical or mental health of your existing children, or that your life would be at risk.

The law in Scotland is slightly different, but works in much the same way as in England and Wales. It is much more strict in Northern Ireland, which is why many women from Northern Ireland come to England to have an abortion.

Abortions are supposed to be available free on the NHS, but NHS abortions are rarely performed after twelve weeks (i.e. twelve weeks from the beginning of your last period) and are often hard to obtain. About half the abortions in Great Britain are carried out through private agencies, partly because they offer a quicker service.

Do I have to see my GP?

It is a good idea to talk things over with your GP as, if you want an NHS abortion, your GP will have to refer you to a local hospital. There you would be seen by another doctor who has to agree that you qualify for an abortion, and that he or she or one of his or her staff will do it. You would then be given an appointment for the operation. Your GP can also refer you to one of the private agencies (see below). However, you do not have to go through your GP – you can approach one of these agencies direct.

What if my GP refuses to help?

If your GP has religious or moral objections to abortion, you should ask to be referred to a colleague. If you have made up your mind that you want an abortion, do not be bamboozled by delaying tactics, like coming back after a few weeks to see if you have missed another period. Ask for an immediate referral, or contact one of the private agencies yourself.

Private agencies

If you are going to have an abortion done privately, it is probably best to go to one of the non-profit-making charities which carry out abortions. (See pages 93–97.)

There are also a number of commercial abortion agencies, which, like the charities, are controlled by DHSS regulations, but their prices are usually higher than those charged by the non-profit-making agencies. These are:

The British Pregnancy Advisory Service The BPAS has around twenty full or part-time branches throughout Britain, and five nursing homes which carry out abortions at Bournemouth, Brighton, Doncaster, Leamington Spa and Liverpool.

The Pregnancy Advisory Service and *Marie Stopes House* also have their own nursing homes. Although both are London-based, they see women from all over the country.

The Brook Advisory Centres There are twenty-one of these centres for young people and, although they do not carry out abortions, they can offer counselling and advice and refer you either for an NHS abortion, or to a private agency.

What will it cost?

NHS abortions are free. Outside the NHS prices vary slightly. At PAS, for instance, it currently costs £35 for a consultation, plus £160 for the operation, provided your pregnancy is thirteen weeks or less.

At BPAS, prices start at £156 for an early abortion. If money is a problem, the charities will do what they can to help. Most have some kind of easy payment scheme, so that you do not have to pay all the money before you have the abortion.

What if I have not yet made up my mind?

All the agencies above will help you to come to a decision if you are unsure. They will not put pressure on you to have an abortion if this is not really what you want. If you think you would rather continue with the pregnancy, but are unsure how you would manage, then *LIFE* offers telephone advice and non-abortion counselling. If you are single, then another organisation which may be able to help is the *National Council for One Parent Families*. (See pages 95–96.)

27

The *Family Planning Information Service* publishes a useful helpsheet *Unplanned Pregnancy*, which outlines your choices, explains about pregnancy tests, offers advice on where to go for help, and describes what happens during the operation and afterwards. (See page 95.)

AIDS

In theory, all sexually active women, who are not in a one-to-one relationship, are at risk from the AIDS virus. So far, in practice, only a small number of women in Britain have been infected with HIV: blood tests on women attending a clinic for genito-urinary disease at the West London Hospital in 1987, for instance, showed that seven out of about 3,000 were infected with the virus.

In addition, many of the women who are known to be infected are in the high-risk categories – either they or their partners are intravenous drug users, or their partners are bisexual.

However, while some experts believe that the risk to women is low, other experts argue that we cannot afford to be complacent, pointing out that although the spread of the virus into the heterosexual community appears slow, this was also the original pattern in the homosexual community.

Either way, it seems sensible to say that any woman who has more than one sexual partner, or who has a partner who may not be monogamous, should practise safe sex.

If there is any reason for you to suppose you may have contracted the virus, you can have a blood test – this can be done at a clinic for sexually transmitted diseases, called a Special Clinic. You should be counselled first, and the counsellors may try to persuade you against the test if they feel you are very unlikely to have been at any risk.

In any case, a negative result does not always mean you are in the clear. The test detects antibodies, rather than the virus itself, and it can take up to three months (very occasionally longer than this) after the virus has first entered the body, for the body to produce these antibodies. So a negative result does not guarantee that you have *not* been exposed to infection.

There are arguments for and against widespread testing for the HIV virus. The *Terrence Higgins Trust* produces a number of helpful leaflets, including *HIV Antibody: To test or not to test?* and *Women and Aids*.

They can also offer help and advice, not only to AIDS victims, but also to women who have relatives or friends with AIDS. (See page 97.)

ALCOHOL

More women drink alcohol these days, so it is not surprising that more women have drink problems. In the UK, alcoholism is the third greatest killer after heart disease and cancer.

Women are now being advised not to drink alcohol before conception or during pregnancy, or, at any rate, to cut their consumption right down. However, while many of us are aware that alcohol may pose some risks to an unborn child, the message, that women cannot drink as much as men without risking their own health, still has not got through to us all. Whether we like it or not, it seems there are important differences in the way women's bodies can cope with alcohol.

Where to turn for help

Of course, if you are worried about the effects of your drinking on your health, you can make an appointment to see your GP. However, there are also other organisations you could turn to. (See pages 93–96.)

Accept is a national charity which can put you in touch with one of its own branches, or a variety of other services, for a range of counselling and treatment. Accept also operates a *National Drinkwatcher Network* of groups, clubs and local self-help services which can educate people about sensible drinking habits, and may be appropriate for anyone who has a mild drink problem.

Alcohol Concern publishes some useful literature, including a leaflet called *Women and Alcohol*.

Alcoholics Anonymous is a worldwide fellowship of men and women who help each other to stay sober. In Great Britain there are more than 2,000 local groups, meeting usually once or twice a week. Most towns and cities will have an AA listing for a group or central office in the telephone directory.

If you have difficulty in finding a group near you, you can contact the AA General Service Office.

In London the *Alcohol Recovery Project* has four drop-in/advice centres which aim to help people who want to get their drinking under control or give it up altogether. One of these centres, in Islington, is for women only.

BACK PAIN

Given that the bulk of housework and childcare still falls to women, it is not surprising that many of us suffer from problems with our backs. We lug heavy bags of shopping home, we carry strapping toddlers when they refuse to walk, we move furniture around to clean under it, and many of us have to manage elderly, bedridden relatives as well. No wonder our poor backs sometimes give us merry hell.

Unfortunately, although backache is as common as the common cold, doctors still find it difficult to pinpoint exactly what has gone wrong and which part of your back has been damaged. That said, they know a lot more than they did some years ago when almost any form of backache was said to be lumbago or sciatica.

Where to go for help

Your GP should be the first person to see, particularly if it is your first attack of back pain or if you are in severe pain. If things do not get better after a few weeks of conventional treatment (usually rest and pain killers), your doctor may refer you to a specialist in orthopaedics or rheumatology. Or you may be sent to the physiotherapy department of a hospital for treatment. Some hospital physiotherapists run back care clubs or clinics, to teach people how to take care of their backs.

Alternative therapies

More and more people are now turning to manipulation to sort out their problem backs. If you decide you want to consult an osteopath or a chiropracter, you do not have to see your own GP first, although it would be sensible to do so as it may affect later treatment. Back pain can occasionally be a symptom of a condition for which manipulation would be pointless and perhaps even dangerous.

Other alternative therapies include acupuncture and homoeopathy (see page 91).

30

Living with back pain

Some hospitals run special pain clinics for people who have been in pain for months or years. Your doctor may feel a referral would be helpful, so ask about the possibility.

The Back Pain Association publishes information on the causes and prevention of back pain, and can give you details of the nearest self-help back pain group. (See page 93.)

The British Holistic Medical Association book, *Beating Back Pain* by Dr John Tanner, is a mine of information about prevention and treatment.

BREASTS

Breast cancer is the most common type of cancer from which women suffer. In 1983 – the latest year for which figures are available – there were 23,778 new cases of breast cancer among women. However, the treatment for breast cancer has improved greatly over the past ten years or so, and the sooner the condition is diagnosed and treatment begins, the better are the chances of a successful outcome. Although a national screening service will help in this, it will not do away with the need for women to carry out their own breast examinations regularly.

Self-examination

Ideally, you should examine your breasts once every month, preferably a short time after a period has finished. If you no longer have periods, then check them on the first day of every month. There is no set age when you should start checking your breasts, but it is worth remembering that young breasts tend to be naturally lumpy, and breast cancer is rare in women under thirty. However, the risk increases with age, so regular checks become more important as you grow older.

The more used you get to the way your breasts normally feel, the more likely you are to notice any changes. Look out for lumps, as well as changes in the texture and appearance of both the breasts and the nipples.

You can ask your GP to show you how to do a self-examination, or, if you are not comfortable with this, you can ask the doctors or nurses at a family planning or well woman clinic. They should also have some leaflets available for you to take home to remind yourself of what you were told.

The Women's National Cancer Control Campaign produces some very good literature on breast self-examination. They also have a ten-minute video, which can be hired for £10 plus postage and packing. (See page 96.)

Mammography

Mammography is an X-ray technique for examining the breasts, which can detect early abnormalities even before a lump can be felt. Being able to start treatment earlier than would otherwise have been possible is a positive advantage.

In 1987, it was announced that a free NHS breast screening service was to be set up, offering all women, between the ages of fifty and sixty-four, mammography every three years. However, the WNCCC estimated that this would not be fully set up until 1990.

The idea is to have some kind of computerised recall system, using names garnered from the records of the Family Practitioner Committees. So if you fall into the right age group and are registered with a doctor, you should automatically be given an appointment if there is a screening unit in your area.

If you think you qualify, but have not heard anything, then check with your GP or Community Health Council, to see if there is a local unit. If you are too young to qualify, or if there is no NHS unit, you could pay to have a mammography privately.

BUPA, for instance, offers mammography as part of its well woman screening at its medical centres.

If you have any difficulties in tracking down a centre which offers mammography, then write to the WNCCC, enclosing an s.a.e.

What if I find a lump?

Do not panic! Nine out of ten lumps are not cancer at all – they may be cysts which can be drained, or benign growths which can be removed very easily. However, the sooner you go to see your GP, the better. He or she will either put your mind at rest at once, or see that you get effective treatment as soon as possible.

The GP will examine you first and then, if necessary, will either arrange for further tests to be carried out, or refer you to a specialist at a hospital.

There, you may be given a mammography, and a sample of

the cells from the lump will need to be taken out and examined. If the tests show that you do have breast cancer, then the specialist will probably want to carry out further tests to see if the disease has spread. This will help him or her to decide what treatment would be best for you.

Will I lose my breast?

Breast cancer treatment has come a long way since the days when surgeons frequently carried out radical mastectomies (operations to remove all of the breast and the muscles of the chest wall) as a routine response to breast cancer. It may be possible to remove only the lump, or just a small section of the breast. Radiotherapy or chemotherapy may then be given as a back-up. However, many surgeons do advise mastectomy routinely, so it is worth knowing what the alternatives are in order to be able to discuss them.

Another point worth remembering is this: there are times when it is not possible to tell whether a lump is malignant or not, until it is removed and examined under a microscope. If the answer is yes, some surgeons prefer to carry out any further surgery while the patient is still under anaesthetic. Others arrange a second operation, a few days later, so that they can talk over their proposals and the woman can prepare herself.

If you want to be woken up so that you can talk about the results first, then you must make this clear to the doctor. Have it written into your notes if necessary.

If you are unhappy with what has been proposed, you can go back to your GP and ask to be referred for a second opinion. The original consultant need not be told, although many doctors quite understand why women want another opinion and are happy for them to have this if it puts their minds at rest.

The cancer charity BACUP says: 'No cancer treatment should be delayed too long, but a few days or even a few weeks will not prejudice the outcome with breast cancer.'

A very useful organisation to contact, if you want more information or advice about any aspect of breast care or breast surgery, is the *Breast Care and Mastectomy Association*. They also point out that you do not have to be referred to your nearest local hospital. Some women ask to be sent to well-known places, such as the Royal Marsden or Guy's in London. (See page 94.)

Implants and prostheses

If you do have a mastectomy, you will be given a temporary lightweight foam prosthesis, or artificial breast, to fit into your bra. Once the tenderness has gone, you can choose one for long-term use, and quite a large selection of prostheses are available, free, on the NHS. Some hospitals have specially trained advisors to help you find the one that is best for you, others rely on nurses to help. According to DHSS guidelines, you are entitled to a new prosthesis when your old one shows signs of wear and tear, or if you have lost or gained so much weight that it no longer fits.

If you are under private health care, the cost of a prosthesis may vary from between £70 to £100, although some insurance schemes allow a certain amount towards the first one.

The BCMA can advise about prostheses and provides lists of stockists and fitters, and they point out that even if you have had only a partial mastectomy, there are prostheses available to restore your natural contour.

For women who have had a mastectomy, a possible alternative to wearing a prosthesis is a breast implant. This involves implanting a sac of specially moulded silicone into the space where the breast used to be. Sometimes this can be done immediately after the breast has been removed, but sometimes doctors prefer to wait for up to three years, to make sure there is no recurrence of the tumour.

Not all surgeons are familiar with the techniques of implant surgery, and you may, in any case, prefer to have the procedure carried out by a specialist in plastic surgery.

Although implanting is not always possible, where it is, it can often be carried out successfully many years after the original operation. Nor need your age be a problem; successful implants have been given to women in their seventies.

It is possible to have an implant done under the NHS, but not all surgeons will do this. Some health insurance schemes will cover most of the costs, providing you have cleared it with them first. Occasionally they will pay for reconstruction many years after the first operation.

If you think you may want an implant at some time, you should tell your surgeon before your first operation. He or she may be able to modify the way the operation is carried out.

Normally you do not get a nipple with your 'new' breast, although one can sometimes be constructed. Many women find that a moulded silicon nipple, which sticks to the implant, is better. These are not available on the NHS.

The BMCA can answer many of your questions about implants. They also run a volunteer visitor scheme and can put you in touch with a local woman who has also had breast surgery and has come to terms with her experience.

CANCER

As the *Cancer Information Service* points out: 'Cancer isn't a single disease with a single cause and a single type of treatment. There are more than 200 different kinds of cancer, each with its own name and treatment.'

Two of the diseases which affect women are breast cancer and cervical cancer (see Breasts and Cervical Smears), but women may also suffer from cancer of the ovary or the uterus, as well as any of the other cancers, such as lung cancer (see Smoking), skin cancer, or cancer of the colon.

Obviously, if you have any reason to suspect you may be suffering from some form of cancer, or, indeed, if you have any inexplicable new symptoms which do not clear up or improve in a few days, you should consult your GP, who will carry out an examination and refer you to a specialist for further tests if necessary.

Finding out more about cancer

A great deal of fear and ignorance surrounds the whole topic of cancer. This is why the late Vicky Clement-Jones, herself a doctor and a cancer patient, set up *BACUP* (The British Association of Cancer United Patients).

If you want to find out more about a particular cancer, the screening available, or the type of treatment involved, you can write to BACUP's *Cancer Information Service*, or ring the team of specially trained cancer nurses. They can explain what is involved, for instance, if a doctor is talking about surgery, radiotherapy or chemotherapy. (See page 94.)

They will also be able to put you in touch with local support groups and give you information about practical problems, such as getting a mortgage after you have had cancer, or a grant for financial help while you are having cancer treatment.

They can also tell you about the Macmillan and Marie Curie nurses, who are specially trained to look after people with cancer in their own homes, and will suggest ways of exploring the possibility of this kind of care if it is appropriate.

More than twenty leaflets and booklets on different types of cancer and their treatment, as well as tips on coping, are available free from BACUP, and they are also trying to develop a face-to-face counselling service for people who find it hard to talk about their problems on the telephone.

Another useful source of help and information is *Cancer-Link*, a national organisation which operates a network of local groups providing emotional and practical support for cancer sufferers and their families and friends. (See page 94.)

Alternative therapies

Both BACUP and CancerLink deal mainly with orthodox approaches to cancer. However, some people believe that alternative therapies may have a part to play alongside ortho-dox medicine. Alternative practitioners take the view that cancer is not just a disease of the body's cells, but of the whole person and so should be tackled 'holistically'.

Methods used may include meditation and visualisation techniques, diet, psychotherapy and spiritual healing. To find out more about holistic treatment, and where to get it, contact *New Approaches to Cancer*. They can provide information about counsellors, groups and residential centres. (See page 96.)

There are currently around seven or eight residential centres, each with a slightly different approach. The most famous is probably the Bristol *Cancer Help Centre*. Before the Cancer Help Centre accepts patients, they send out an introductory leaflet explaining their programme and the fees charged. If people are still interested, they send for the information pack, which includes the book *The Bristol Programme* by Penny Brohn, and a cassette tape. (The book is also on sale through bookshops.) (See page 94.)

At the time of writing, a five-day residential stay costs £475, plus an extra £124 if another adult accompanies you. A day visit costs £75 initially, plus another £15 for each return visit. However, in dire need there is a bursary fund which may be able to subsidise day visits, and, if you are on supplementary benefit, the DHSS will contribute up to £170 a week towards the cost of a residential stay.

It is necessary to do some homework before deciding to join a programme of the kind offered at Bristol. As they say: 'You must be committed or else you are wasting your time and money – and taking up a place that someone else could be desperate for.'

It is also worth noting that the Cancer Help Centre never claims to 'cure' cancer, but they do claim that they can help you to get the most out of your hospital treatment, may teach you how to avoid unnecessary side-effects from cancer treatments, and will give you a better quality of life.

Cervical smears

Cancer of the cervix can be prevented from developing, or successfully cured, if it is caught early enough. This is why cervical smear testing is so important.

According to DHSS guidelines, women between the ages of twenty and sixty-four should have a smear test every five years, and health authorities have been instructed to set up a call and recall testing system, which the Department of Health is confident will be fully operational by spring 1988.

The aim is to tighten up the screening net – in the past, women, who were not going to their GP or a family planning clinic for contraceptive advice, often slipped through.

Many experts believe, however, that a five-year gap between smear tests is too long, and argue that a three-year gap is better. Also, now that there is evidence that a more virulent form of the disease can affect younger women, they argue that there is a case for starting screening two years after a woman becomes sexually active (while she may still be under twenty) followed by biennial or annual tests for the under-thirties.

How to get a cervical smear test

In theory, if you are between twenty and sixty-four, you should automatically be given an appointment every five years. However, if for some reason the system is not operating in your part of the country, or if you agree with the experts who think women should be tested every three years, ask your GP or local well woman or family planning clinic.

These tests are free. If you are still unable to get one, there are a number of private organisations where you can pay for the test to be carried out.

At most of the BPAS branches, for instance, you can arrange to have the test done for a fee of £10. The Brook Advisory Centres also offer cervical smear tests to clients.

The Women's National Cancer Control Campaign produces some literature on cervical screening, can provide speakers, and has a video called *Test in Time*, which can be hired for £10 plus postage and packing. They can also arrange to set up workplace screening, providing a mobile unit if necessary.

Can I be seen by a woman doctor?

Many women feel uneasy about being examined by a male doctor, and if you would rather be seen by a woman, then say so. Staff at family planning clinics, surgeries and health centres are often asked this and will usually try to be helpful. In any case, you can always ask for a nurse to be present in the surgery while a doctor is looking at you.

What happens next?

If the test shows that your cervix is healthy, you may not be told. For your own peace of mind, you might like to ring for confirmation that your test was all right.

Sometimes you will be asked to have another smear test done. This may simply be because not enough cells were collected to enable the lab technician to complete the test. Or there may appear to be minor changes in some of the cells – the doctor will then probably want you to have two further smears, at intervals of six months, just to make sure your cervix is really healthy. Mild abnormalities of this kind can return to normal without any treatment at all.

If you are asked to have another smear and this still shows abnormal cells, your doctor will either arrange for further tests, or you will be referred directly to a hospital specialist. This does not mean you *have* cancer, but if the abnormal cells are left untreated, they may *develop* into cancer.

Some hospitals will have the facilities for culposcopy (the use of an instrument, rather like a small microscope, to examine the cervix), which is usually done at an out-patient clinic. If this is not available, a cone biopsy will be done, combining treatment and diagnosis. This is a small operation, carried out under general anaesthetic, and will mean a short stay in hospital.

The other main treatments are laser therapy, cryotherapy, cold coagulation (all done in a hospital out-patient clinic) and diathermy (carried out under general anaesthetic and involving a short stay in hospital).

The kind of treatment you will be offered will depend on a number of factors, including the facilities available at your local hospital. If you want to know more about types of treatment, or about cervical cancer, then BACUP has some useful booklets and their Cancer Information Service, which is staffed by fully trained cancer nurses, should be able to help. (See page 94.)

New techniques

Experts have been working on a number of ways of improving the accuracy and efficiency of cervical screening – one of the problems is that the more women who come for screening, the longer they must all wait, both for appointments and results.

One new technique involves taking a photograph of the cervix, rather than a sample of cells, which can then be examined by a gynaecologist after it has been magnified several times. This technique can be used instead of a repeat smear, if the first test appears to show a problem. At the time of writing, this is available on the NHS at only one London hospital, the Royal Northern, for an experimental period, and also at the Marie Stopes clinic in London, where the service, including a cervigram and smear, costs £41.

Marie Stopes are hoping to extend the service to their centres in Leeds and Manchester.

National Survey on Cervical Cancer

In late 1983, the subject of cervical cancer screening was widely discussed. The opinions of the Department of Health, medical organisations, health authorities and experts of all sorts were being sought and published. Occasionally individual women, famous and unknown, were asked for their comments on the screening programme, but there seemed to be no real attempt to discover how women in general reacted to and were involved in cervical cancer screening. Given that the success of this preventative health care measure stands or falls by its success in reaching women, the National Federation of Women's Institutes and the Women's National Cancer Control Campaign proposed that the two organisations should work together to establish the extent of women's knowledge of the system and how appropriate it was to their needs.

In order to do this, several things had to be established:
● What women knew about cervical cancer.
● What anxieties women had about cervical smear tests.

39

- What women knew about the screening programme in terms of sources of testing and frequency.
- What women thought about the screening programme in general.

Results of the survey
- Although the majority of women replying had been smear tested, there were still many misconceptions about the purpose of the test. There is clearly a need for better education and information.
- Two of the major concerns to emerge from the survey were the recall system, and the fact that the results of the tests were not automatically made available. 68 per cent of the women had never received any form of reminder.
- The majority of WI members questioned would prefer to see a three-year interval between tests – rather than the five-year one currently recommended by the DHSS.
- Embarrassment about internal examinations and reluctance to be tested by a male doctor affected many women. The survey showed a need for more reassurance and encouragement on the part of medical staff. 65 per cent of the women stated that a smear test had never been suggested by a doctor.
- Many women – especially those living in rural areas – faced transport problems in attending for tests. There were also difficulties in discovering where and when to go for tests. The survey revealed a need for more well woman clinics – over 62 per cent would prefer to have the test carried out at such a clinic.

CONTRACEPTION

Family planning services are provided free of charge on the NHS for anyone normally resident in the United Kingdom, regardless of age, sex or marital status.

The services are confidential and available from hospitals, clinics and most family doctors. Supplies are also free, either direct from a clinic or on prescription, although GPs cannot prescribe condoms.

As a result of cutbacks within the health services, there may be some restrictions on supplies at clinics. Limits on supplies per person per year have always existed, but now that budgets are being squeezed, these may be more rigorously applied. For instance, no more than twelve condoms a month may be supplied to any one person, and only two caps a year (although this last figure should be sufficient in most cases).

There are three types of contraception available: barrier methods, such as condoms, or sheaths, and the cap, or diaphragm, often used in conjunction with spermicidal creams; various kinds of contraceptive pill; or sterilisation. You should also be able to get advice about natural family planning methods (see below). Sponges containing spermicide are not available at family planning clinics, but can be bought over the counter at chemists.

The GP

Most GPs give free family planning and will describe all the methods to you, counsel you as to the best method, and prescribe the one you choose. Your doctor can send you elsewhere if you want a particular service he or she does not give – some GPs, for instance, do not fit IUDs. However, if you wish to use condoms, you will be unable to get these through your GP, although family planning clinics can prescribe them.

When it comes to the various types of contraceptive pill, spermicidal creams or pessaries, or the cap, you will be given a prescription to take to a chemist, and you will pay no charges for these supplies.

If your own GP does not provide family planning services, or if, for any reason, you prefer not to discuss birth control with your own doctor, you are entitled to go to another GP for this service. Some GPs provide birth control for patients who see a different GP for general health care.

Lists of GPs are available in libraries and from your local Family Practitioner Committee, whose address will be on your medical card or in the local telephone directory. Those doctors who give contraceptive advice are identified by the letter C after their names.

About 60 per cent of women go to their GP, rather than to a clinic, for birth control. In some cases, this may be because there is little real choice. Recent cutbacks in the health service have led to the closure of a number of family planning clinics, and parts of the country now have none at all. Some clinics may hold just one or two sessions a week, at inconvenient times. It may also be difficult to reach a clinic if you do

41

not live near a town or city, and your GP's surgery may be nearer.

The family planning clinic

There are just under 2,000 free family planning clinics in the UK. Clinics used to be run by the Family Planning Association on a fee-paying basis, until 1974/75, when they were taken over by the NHS, and they now come under the umbrella of the various health authorities. Some are still held in the out-patients departments of hospitals, although nowadays they are more commonly to be found in health centres.

The quickest way to track down your nearest family planning clinic is probably to ring your local health centre. An alternative would be to look under Family Planning in your local telephone directory.

If you have any difficulties, the Family Planning Information Service keeps a list of clinics.

Women who go to clinics often do so because they feel confident that they are being seen by family planning experts. As Ellen Bingham, an information officer of the FPA says: 'Unless GPs are particularly interested in the subject you can't expect them to be totally up to date. Many women feel they get a better quality of care at a clinic.'

Another reason why some women prefer to go to a clinic is that you can ask to see a woman doctor if you wish.

What happens at a clinic?

At your first appointment you are usually seen, initially, by a nurse, who will take a case history and carry out a routine examination. She will check your weight and your blood pressure and ask you questions about your menstrual cycle and gynaecological history, so it helps if you go with the date of your last period, and any other relevant information, at your fingertips. She will also ask what forms of contraception you are currently using.

Your notes will then be passed to the doctor, who will talk to you in more detail and help you to choose the form of birth control to suit you. Depending on the form of contraception used, you will be asked to return for a follow-up visit every three, six or twelve months.

Will my GP be told?

It is best if your family doctor knows if you are going to take the pill, have an IUD fitted, or be sterilised. In most cases the clinic doctor will write to your GP – but if you do not want this to happen, then you should make this clear.

Contraceptives and younger women

As the law stands, if a doctor believes a girl under the age of sixteen is at risk of pregnancy, and he or she counsels her accordingly, she can be provided with contraceptives without her parents being informed. However, the *Brook Centres*, which offer free birth control advice and supplies to young people, reported that, after the Gillich rulings, fewer clients were willing to let them inform GPs about their visit, presumably because they were afraid confidentiality would be broken.

They stress that, while they welcome parents and liaison with GPs, they do offer a confidential service and you do not have to wait until you are sixteen if you need their help. There are now twenty-one centres throughout the country. To find your nearest one, contact the central office. (See page 94.)

In fact, all family planning clinics and GPs offer all women – regardless of age – a confidential service. So although a doctor might encourage a girl to talk to her parents, or might, indeed, refuse to prescribe contraception for her unless she did, he or she would not feel obliged to tell anyone about her visit or request.

Domiciliary service

If you are housebound for some reason – because you have a very young baby, or if you are disabled – you may be able to get help in your own home. Someone, usually a health visitor or a nurse, will visit you to talk about contraception and to provide supplies. To arrange this, you would have to contact your own GP, health visitor, midwife or social worker.

Private clinics

Of course, there are a number of clinics outside the health service, which offer contraceptive services among other things. The Brook Advisory Centres, mentioned above, cater mainly for the under-thirties. The *British Pregnancy Advisory Service*, a non-profit-making charity, has about twenty

43

branches around the country, and currently charges £15, plus the cost of supplies, for two visits a year. (See page 94.)

Emergency measures – the morning-after pill or IUD

No matter how much care you take about contraception, sometimes things go wrong.

- Condoms burst, a stomach upset may mean the pill does not get absorbed, you may even realise, belatedly, that you forgot to take the pill at all.
- You may simply not have been prepared for intercourse – at least half the episodes of first-time intercourse are un-protected, and many more first-time lovers use inadequate precautions, as do couples reuniting after a period of separation.
- You may have been raped.

Under these kinds of emergencies, free post-coital (more commonly called 'morning-after') contraception should be available.

The popular term is somewhat misleading. There are two types of post-coital contraception: two special doses of a high-strength combined pill, and the fitting of an IUD. The pills work if treatment is started up to seventy-two hours after intercourse, the IUD if fitted within five days. The IUD can be left in place if you decide this method of birth control is suitable for you.

Where to go

In theory, you should be able to get the morning-after pill from your GP or local family planning clinic, although in practice you may find it easier to get an urgent appointment with your own doctor than the clinic, and the time factor is crucial. For that reason, it may be harder to get an IUD fitted, as many GPs do not carry out this procedure.

If you have any problems, telephone one of the private or charitable organisations which offer a post-coital service, to find out whether there is a clinic near you. These include the *Brook Advisory Centres*, the *British Pregnancy Advisory Service*, the *Pregnancy Advisory Service* and *Marie Stopes*. At BPAS, for instance, you would normally pay £15 for post-coital con-traception, but this would include follow-up visits and con-traceptive care for a year. (See pages 93–97.)

Natural family planning

Some women are unhappy about using barrier or hormonal methods of contraception, and prefer to use 'natural' techniques. For others, these may be the only techniques which fit in with their religious or moral beliefs.

There are various ways of identifying the 'safe' period: the temperature method, the Billings or mucus method, the calendar method, and a combination of methods. Each method relies on a woman's ability to identify her fertile phase so that she can avoid intercourse at a time when pregnancy would be likely.

Where to go

Your GP or local family planning clinic should be able to help you, and you can get free fertility thermometers and booklets for recording temperatures from them, but it is better to be taught by someone who specialises in these techniques. You can contact the *Natural Family Planning Service*, run by the Catholic Marriage Advisory Council, who have booklets on the method and can put you in touch with a tutor.

Alternatively, you could contact the *Natural Family Planning Centre*. (See page 96.)

Sterilisation

Once you have decided that you have all the children you want, you may opt for sterilisation, either for yourself or your partner (this is normally called a vasectomy). For women, the operation is usually done under a general anaesthetic and involves admission to a hospital or nursing home. For men, in most cases, a local anaesthetic will be used and they will be treated on an out-patient basis, going home after a short rest.

The NHS provides sterilisation for both men and women, and your GP will be able to advise and refer you. However, waiting lists may be long in some areas. Sterilisation can be carried out privately. At BPAS, for instance, the operation currently costs £176 for women and £75 for men.

Sterilisation should always be thought of as a permanent step. However, there may be reasons why some people decide they would like to try to have the process reversed – perhaps if they have a new partner, or a child has died. As always within the NHS, waiting lists vary – as do success rates. At BPAS (where a vasectomy reversal costs £530 and a sterilisation reversal £935) they say that about 50 per cent of couples have achieved pregnancy after vasectomy reversal. For women, they say, rates vary from 30 to 70 per cent, depending on the way the original sterilisation was carried out.

CYSTITIS

Eight out of ten women suffer from cystitis at some time in their lives. For many women it is only a matter of an isolated attack or two, but for others the condition can return over and over again.

What to do

The first thing you should do is collect a urine sample and give this to your GP as soon as possible, so that it can be analysed in case you have some kind of infection that can be treated. It is worth noting that if you cannot get to your GP, you can always present yourself at the nearest Special Clinic, the clinic which deals with sexually transmitted diseases, even though cystitis is not a sexually transmitted disease (although sexual intercourse may trigger off an attack). The doctors there will see you, particularly if you say you think you have some kind of discharge.

Self-help

Even before you see a doctor, you should try some immediate self-help remedies.
- At the first signs, increase your fluid intake. Aim to drink half a pint (quarter litre) of water every twenty minutes for the first three hours.
- Take a teaspoon of bicarbonate of soda in water every hour for three hours. If you cannot stand the taste, mix it with honey.
- Take two mild painkillers.
- Lie down, put your feet up and try to relax. Keep warm and put a hot water bottle on your back or pelvic area.

Most doctors routinely prescribe antibiotics, but many attacks of cystitis are not caused by infections. If you suffer from repeated attacks then it would be worth tracking down a copy of *Understanding Cystitis, A complete self-help guide* by Angela Kilmartin. Mrs Kilmartin (see page 95) may be able to put you in touch with a local self-help group, and she also counsels sufferers. She charges £10 an hour.

DRUGS

Few of us can say we never take drugs – the odd swig of cough mixture; an aspirin for a headache. Used properly, drugs can make a great difference to our lives. But there are some conditions which do not respond to drugs, so we should not expect to come out of the surgery with a prescription every time we visit the doctor.

Pharmacists

Pharmacists are trained to know about drugs and medicines. It is their job to supply whatever your doctor has prescribed and to make sure you know how to take it. If you are not sure, ask. They also sell various medicines which can be obtained without a prescription, so if you have a minor problem, it is a good idea to seek their advice about what to take. If you want information about medicines and your local pharmacist cannot help, you can contact *The Pharmaceutical Society of Great Britain*. (See page 96.)

Prescriptions

Prescription charges are now a fact of life, and you will have to pay a charge for each item on your prescription unless you are exempt, or have been prescribed contraceptives, which are free. If you are going to need a lot of prescriptions, you can buy a 'season ticket', which should save you some money. You will need the relevant form, which is available from your GP, your pharmacist or your local DHSS office.

Some women pay when they need not. Full-time students under nineteen, for example, are exempt, as are women over sixty, pregnant women, or women with a baby less than a year old. The same applies to women on supplementary benefit or family income supplement. And if you are on a low income, but not getting supplementary benefit (as an older, full-time student perhaps) you may also qualify for exemption. Check it out with your local DHSS office. Their number and address will be in the telephone directory.

If you are being treated privately (or if your GP prescribes something which the NHS has not specified it will supply), then you will have to pay the full cost yourself. This will include the cost of the drug, the dispensing fee and a small charge for the bottle or jar.

Questions to ask your doctor

A study published in the *British Medical Journal* showed that more than two-thirds of those prescribed drugs showed little interest in what they had been given. Only 28 per cent asked about side-effects and only 32 per cent asked what the drug did.

But it is in your own interest to know what you are taking and how it might make you feel. These are some of the questions you might ask your doctor.

● What kind of pills are these? What are they supposed to do and how will I know if they are working or not?
● How should I take them? How important are they – and what might happen if I stop taking them?
● Do they have side-effects?
● Can I drive/drink alcohol/take other medicines while I am taking them?
● How long should I carry on taking them and what should I do with any pills I don't need?
● Will I need to see you again and, if so, what will you want to know?

Emergencies

There should always be one pharmacy in your area open late. It may not always be the same one – the local press should carry details and there will also be a notice in all the local pharmacies, giving the hours and rota times.

Any prescriptions marked 'urgent' by your doctor can be made up, during the night or on public holidays, by a pharmacist who is on a special list, which is supplied to the police and emergency services.

If the worst comes to the worst, you can contact your local police station for this information. The pharmacist may insist that a police officer is present before he or she opens the shop and, even then, can refuse to attend, although this rarely happens.

Addiction

Drugs can make us better – or they can make things worse. It is a sad fact that many people become addicted to drugs of one sort or another. So what should you do if you think you need help, either for yourself or because a friend or a relative has drug problems?

Some GPs are very knowledgeable about drug addiction, while others know very little. Attitudes towards addicts can vary considerably too. If you approach your doctor, it is likely that you will be referred to the nearest rehabilitation centre.

There are ways of finding out yourself what treatment is available. Your local library, *Citizen's Advice Bureau* and the *Samaritans* will all have a copy of a directory produced by the *Standing Conference on Drug Abuse* (SCODA). This directory is called *Drug Problems: Where To Get Help*, and it lists all the known drug services in the United Kingdom.

You can also dial the operator and ask for *Freephone Drug Problems*. You will then hear a recorded message giving a series of telephone numbers for each of the English counties, and other numbers to call if you come from Scotland, Wales or Northern Ireland. Have a piece of paper and a pen handy before you ring.

The drug service listed for your county may not be the nearest one to you, but the people there will be able to refer you on to an agency or centre that would suit your needs.

According to David Turner, director of SCODA, the provision of services for people with drug problems varies throughout the country. In some parts there is a good network of service; elsewhere it is patchy.

The vast majority of services, from residential drug rehabilitation centres to hospital clinics or drug centres, are free, but a few may ask for a contribution or make a charge of some kind. Most of the services are oversubscribed.

Private services are also available – *Broadway Lodge* at Weston-super-Mare, for instance has been called the Eton of rehabilitation houses. But, says David Turner, it is an idea to talk over the problem first so that you can sort out your needs, and only then decide what kind of service is appropriate. (See page 94.)

Another source of information is *Release*. This is a national, alternative, legal and welfare organisation, which can advise and refer drug users, their friends and relatives. Release can also help with drug-related legal problems and there is a national twenty-four-hour emergency telephone line. (See page 96.)

Two other organisations which may prove helpful are *Narcotics Anonymous* (see page 95), a network of self-help groups run by addicts for addicts, along the lines of Alcoholics Anonymous, for the purpose of recovery. *Families Anonymous* (see page 94) helps families and friends of drug-dependent people. (See also Tranquillisers.)

EATING PROBLEMS

From an early age, women are often under a lot of pressure to look attractive – and these days most people assume attractive equals slim. We are constantly bombarded with the message that thin is beautiful, so it is not surprising that a lot of us worry about our weight and the food we eat.

Nor is it surprising, therefore, that many of us also see-saw between eating what we like when we like, one week, and then spending the next seven days on a low-calorie crash diet. Some women even become so obsessive that they develop anorexia nervosa or bulimia.

Diet and nutrition

It need not cost a fortune to eat healthily and sensibly. Your Community Health Council may be able to put you in touch with a community dietician, who can provide information and advice about diet and nutrition in general.

The Health Education Council (see page 95) produces a range of useful leaflets, including *Fibre in your Food*, and *Fat – Who needs it? The British Nutrition Foundation* can also supply some useful literature (see page 94).

Dieting

If you think you need to lose weight, your GP can advise you. Some doctors prescribe appetite-depressant drugs (particularly doctors who run private weight-control clinics), but most do not, because as soon as a course is finished, the appetite – and the weight – tend to come back. These drugs may also be addictive.

In extreme cases of obesity, it is possible that you will be referred to a hospital specialist. And, in rare cases, surgery may be used to remove excess weight.

There are all kinds of diets and diet aids around today. Before you embark on any, it might be a good idea to find a copy of the book *Which? Way To Slim*. It gives a very thorough run-down on the various approaches to slimming. You should also check with your doctor before you try any self-help measures.

It is worth noting that most of today's experts say that the best way to lose weight and keep it off is not by reducing your calorie intake to a minimum, but through exercise.

Anorexia, bulimia and compulsive eating

If you think your eating habits are really out of hand, you should seek medical help. Generally, a GP will persuade a woman suffering from anorexia nervosa or bulimia to go into hospital (often to the psychiatric wing) where her intake of food will be supervised by experienced doctors and nurses. She may also be involved in some kind of psychotherapy, and this will probably continue once she is well enough to be discharged.

One organisation which offers information and support to sufferers and their families is *Anorexic Aid*. They also co-ordinate a network of self-help groups so that anorexics can share their problems and learn how others managed to overcome similar difficulties. (See page 93.)

Unfortunately, not all GPs are as sensitive in their approach towards eating disorders as they might be. In addition, many anorexics, for example, will not seek medical help.

The Women's Therapy Centre runs workshops for women with eating disorders. If you are not London-based, then they may be able to put you in touch with someone locally who can counsel or help, or refer you to a self-help group. They also have useful leaflets on bulimia and compulsive eating, which cost £2 each. (See page 97.)

GYNAECOLOGICAL PROBLEMS

There are a number of gynaecological conditions which may give rise to symptoms such as heavy, painful or irregular periods, or pain during intercourse. Many women put up with things like this for a long time, either because they fear that their doctors will be unsympathetic, or because they are frightened to find out if something is wrong. Some simply find anything like this embarrassing to talk about.

It is important to see a doctor if there is something worrying you. Do not suffer in silence. If there is something wrong, the sooner it is put right, the better. Go to see your GP, who will probably examine you and then refer you to a consultant gynaecologist for further investigation and treatment if necessary.

Your GP may have a good idea what is causing the problem, but the necessary facilities may not be available in your local hospital for confirming this diagnosis.

Fibroids, for example, can be diagnosed by X-ray, ultrasound or an exploratory operation. Endometriosis can only be confirmed by a laparoscopy or surgical exploration. Ovarian cysts can often be felt during a pelvic examination, and their presence is then confirmed by ultrasound.

Pelvic inflammatory disease, the umbrella term used by doctors to describe any infection and inflammation of the pelvic organs, can sometimes be difficult to diagnose. Symptoms include fever, pain in the lower abdomen, vaginal discharge, pain on intercourse and heavy, painful periods. PID can flare up very quickly, or the infection may lie dormant for some time. Some women find they have recurring attacks.

If you think you have PID, rather than making an appointment with your GP, you could consider going to a Special Clinic for sexually transmitted diseases (check the telephone directory under Venereal Diseases if you do not know where your local clinic is) as they will be able to test for infection straightaway.

What if I'm still worried or don't understand what I've been told?

Do not be afraid to ask as many questions as you need to. If, even after this, you are still confused or alarmed, then there are two sources of information and advice which you might find useful.

Women's Health Concern answers enquiries about gynaecological problems (see page 97; s.a.e.s please).

The Women's Health Information Centre can also provide information. (See page 97.)

Self-help groups

If you suffer from a particular condition, you might be able to find a self-help group. Check with your local library or Community Health Council.

For instance, *The Endometriosis Society* (see page 94) provides counselling for sufferers and also produces an information pack. The society can give you details of self-help groups, and meetings and regular workshop days are held in London. (See also Menopause; Hysterectomy; PMS.)

HYSTERECTOMY

If you have been told you need a hysterectomy, it may be of little comfort to know that it is a very common operation – around 1,000 are carried out in Britain each week.

A hysterectomy may be done for one of a number of reasons, ranging from cancer to period problems, but although the operation is common enough, many women find themselves facing it with little or no discussion beforehand about why it needs to be done, what exactly will happen, or how they might feel afterwards.

Some hospitals have booklets which they give to patients when they are admitted for the operation. Many more do not and, in any case, most women would feel happier if they were given as much information as possible before this stage.

Is a hysterectomy always necessary?

Unless cancer is involved, there may be alternative treatments for your problems. Nikki Henriques and Anne Dickson say, in their book *Women on Hysterectomy*, which is well worth reading: 'Fibroids can be removed by myomectomy; a prolapsed womb can be repaired; endometriosis, heavy bleeding and PMS can be relieved with hormonal medication or even herbal rememdies.'

They also point out that age can be another important factor – if you have fibroids and are close to the menopause the fibroids may shrink and the symptoms disappear as your natural oestrogen level falls.

Sometimes, too, heavy bleeding and other conditions linked to PMS may be stress-related, so tackling the stressful areas of your life, rather than having surgery, might be a better solution. However, as Henriques and Dickson say, whether alternative treatments will be effective or not will depend on how severe your symptoms are.

What questions to ask

If you do not have cancer and there is no urgent need for you to have a hysterectomy, the first person you need to question is yourself. How will you feel about losing your womb? Do you associate it with your own sense of femininity and sexuality? Will it matter if you cannot have children?

How incapacitating are your symptoms? Are they merely inconvenient or are they really ruining your enjoyment of life?

Women who have sensitive GPs may be given the opportunity of exploring these issues early on. Others may be referred to gynaecologists prepared to counsel and advise. But this is far from routine.

Whatever else your GP does or does not do, he or she should refer you to someone who has a good reputation, rather than leaving it to chance and the vaguaries of how the waiting lists are organised at the local hospital. GPs do get some feedback from former hysterectomy cases, and can also make some enquiries on the medical grapevine. Ask who will be treating you and what they are like.

It always helps if you go to an appointment – either with a GP or a consultant – armed with notes to remind you of the questions you would like answered. When you see the consultant, it is also a good idea to ask specific questions about the kind of hysterectomy he or she is proposing to do.

To some extent, this will depend on the condition of your cervix, ovaries and uterus, but most surgeons have their own preferences, too.

What exactly will be removed – your cervix, ovaries and Fallopian tubes, or just your uterus? The most commonly held medical view these days is that it is best to leave the ovaries in place whenever possible, so that they can continue to produce natural hormones. If the ovaries are removed before the menopause has occurred naturally, then you will experience an artificial menopause. If this happens a long time before nature intended, the symptoms usually associated with the menopause may be severe. HRT (hormone replacement therapy) may be prescribed to help, but not all doctors are in favour of this. (See HRT.)

Will you be left with a scar down the centre of your stomach, or will you have a bikini-line scar? Or will the operation be done vaginally (technically the most difficult way), which leaves no scar at all? Will your skin be clipped together or sewn up? Will you be routinely catheterised?

Support and self-help

You could contact *Women's Health Concern* (see page 97) if you need advice or information. The *Wirral Hysterectomy Support Group* (see page 97) is an organisation which will try to put you in touch with counsellors near you, who have themselves experienced hysterectomy. Please send an s.a.e.

INFERTILITY

It can be heartbreaking if you want a baby, but just cannot seem to get pregnant. Yet infertility is not an uncommon problem – indeed, many experts believe it is becoming more common for a number of reasons. These include: decreased fertility in those who delay starting a family until they are in their thirties; an increase in sexually transmitted diseases; a few people are affected by prolonged use of the pill or abortion; even the effects of drugs and pollutants.

Modern techniques have improved the chances for childless couples to have the baby they long for, but it is still a sad fact that even the best of modern medicine cannot help everyone. That said, there are steps you can take to help yourself, and a number of ways in which you may be able to get help from the medical profession.

Self-help measures

Assuming that you have got the basics right (that is to say, you are having vaginal intercourse and your partner is ejaculating sperm inside your vagina), there are some simple steps to take, which can improve your chances of conceiving.

These include the timing of love-making (knowing when you are ovulating and when it is best to make love), the positions to use, and tips like not getting up or washing after intercourse, and avoiding lubricating creams and jellies, which can have a spermicidal effect.

Your GP or family planning clinic doctors will be able to advise you, and may be able to teach you techniques for charting your monthly cycle, using basal body temperature and/or cervical mucus observations. You can also get information from the *Natural Family Planning Service* or the *Natural Family Planning Centre* (see Contraception). *The Family Planning Information Service* has a helpsheet, *Planning a Pregnancy*. (See pages 93–97.)

A newer way of working out your fertility window is by using the dipsticks you can buy over the counter at a pharmacy. These are not cheap, however, and it is probably a better idea to get to know your own body and its cycle.

Other things which may help are losing weight (both of you), stopping smoking, drinking alcohol and taking drugs of any kind (if you are taking prescribed drugs, do not stop without consulting your doctor first).

Heat changes can affect a man's fertility. Sometimes it helps if the man stops wearing tight-fitting underpants and trousers, although results can take three months to show.

A book which gives a lot of useful self-help advice, and covers the whole subject of infertility thoroughly is *Why Us?* by Dr Andrew Stanway. It is definitely worth getting hold of a copy.

You can also contact *The National Association for the Childless* (see page 96), by writing or telephoning for an information list which will give details of the factsheets available, which cover all aspects of childlessness. These are free if you join (membership is currently £12.50 a year). Otherwise they cost 50p or 60p each.

The Family Planning Information Service produces a help-sheet called *Infertility Tests and Treatment*.

When to seek help

Even when everything is working perfectly, the average time it takes for a couple to conceive is 5.3 months. Only a quarter of couples manage first time. So how long should you wait before you seek help?

Around 75 per cent of couples trying for a baby will achieve pregnancy within a year. Women who have not been taking the pill seem, on average, to get pregnant quicker – around 80 to 90 per cent of this group normally take six months to a year. But the differences level out – after two years, pill-users have the same chance of pregnancy as non-pill-users.

These days most experts suggest that if you have not managed to start a pregnancy within twelve months of normal sex (and without using any form of contraception) then you should seek help. So do not be fobbed off – the sooner you are checked out and treated, if necessary, the better, particularly if you have waited to have a family and are now in your thirties rather than your twenties.

Your GP should be your first call, although some family planning clinics run infertility sessions.

What happens next?

Your GP is likely to refer you to a specialist. According to David Owens, director of the National Association for the Childless, provision for infertility investigation is patchy and, although you may be referred to a specialist clinic, it is possible that you will be dealt with by doctors working in the obstetrics and gynaecology department of a local hospital.

David Owens says that it is better to be referred to a specialist clinic if this is possible, but often the cost, in terms of time and money spent in travelling, rules this out.

Initially, both you and your husband should be interviewed so that a detailed medical history can be taken, and you will both be examined to rule out any obvious medical causes for the problem.

After this a series of tests is likely to be carried out – the doctor concerned will decide which ones should be done when. The idea of the tests is to establish, first of all, that the woman is ovulating, that the sperm are plentiful and healthy, and that they can live in the woman's cervical mucus. Then it may be necessary to make sure that the woman's Fallopian tubes are not blocked, and, if the reason for the couple's infertility is still not clear, more detailed tests, to check your hormonal system, may be necessary.

Doctors still have a lot to learn about fertility, but they know much more than they used to. These days drugs can be used to control ovulation in a much more precise way than before. Microsurgical techniques and *in vitro* fertilisation can offer hope to women with badly damaged Fallopian tubes. Even cases where the woman produces antibodies against her husband's sperm (or where he produces his own) can be detected and treated.

Can we speed things up?

One of the most frustrating things is that all the tests can seem to take so much time. Simply waiting to be seen by a specialist in the first place may involve a period of several months.

It is worth bearing in mind that carrying out tests on a man's sperm can be done easily and should, ideally, be carried out as soon as possible. Infertility is found as often in men as in women.

David Owens also points out that knowing what kind of investigations may be necessary – indeed, understanding as much as possible about infertility and its treatment – can help you to move the processes along politely but firmly. 'If you know the basic ground rules, you can play the game. I'm very much in favour of people knowing as much as possible about what they are going through. For instance, the language used by many doctors is by no means accessible to the layman. That's why we produce our own factsheets.'

It is also a fact of life that if you can afford to pay for treatment privately, you will be able to speed up the process to some extent. Once again, the NAC can, through local self-help groups, let you know if there is someone appropriate to whom you could be referred in your area, and they can also provide a checklist, giving you some idea of what various treatments will cost.

Even so, testing and treatment can take years rather than months and the emotional price can be very high.

Could we have a test-tube baby?

Ever since the birth of Louise Brown in 1978, test-tube babies have made the headlines. But although *in vitro* fertilisation (to give this technique its correct term) is now more widely available, and is offered at about forty centres in Britain, it is still not the answer for many couples.

The majority of the centres only accept private patients, so cost may rule this idea out. Other factors are likely to be taken into account before couples are taken onto waiting lists: factors such as age or the stability of the marriage.

And in any case, IVF may simply not be appropriate. If you are having trouble getting pregnant, do not assume IVF will be the answer to all your prayers. There may be other possibilities – tubal surgery, for instance, or artificial insemination – but in any case, for most couples the basic tests and treatments are all that are necessary.

MENOPAUSE

Menopause literally means the last period, but these days we use the term to cover the years before and after menstruation finally stops. There are still doctors who feel that as menopause is not a life-threatening condition, but a natural process, women should learn to live with hot flushes, vaginal discomfort, dry skin, headaches and the other side-effects that may accompany the change of life. Thankfully, others have a more enlightened attitude.

When should I seek help?

Many women go through the menopause without any problems. Others suffer from hot flushes and so on, but feel able to cope. But if you are at the stage where the symptoms are so severe, or have gone on for so long, that your relationship, your business or your social life is suffering, then you should certainly seek help.

Where to go for help

Most women begin by going to their GP. Some will offer treatment, others will refer women to a consultant gynae-cologist at a hospital, or to a menopause clinic. If your GP is unwilling to refer you, an alternative possibility is to get a referral from your local family planning clinic if there is one.

A few clinics will accept self-referrals. To find out if there is a menopause clinic in your area, you can either ask your GP or contact the Community Health Council. Other sources of information may be *Women's Health Concern* and the *Women's Health Information Centre* (see page 97). You could also ask to be referred by your GP to a private consultant.

Hormone replacement therapy (HRT)

Recently there has been much debate about the use of hormone replacement therapy once the menopause has started. There is no doubt that it helps to prevent osteoporosis – brittle bones – but doctors disagree as to whether, as a result, all women should have it, or just those who might be particularly at risk. Unfortunately, there is no foolproof way of knowing in advance which women these might be.

HRT is also used to treat hot flushes, sweats and vaginal dryness. Many women say it also improves skin tone and gives them a new vitality. However, it cannot be prescribed for everyone and there are risks, although, as always, the experts argue about the extent of these.

If you are interested in HRT, then you can seek help from your GP, or ask to be referred to a specialist. First, however, it is a good idea to learn as much about it as you can. You can contact *The Amarant Trust* (see page 93). The Trust has also started a specialist clinic (staffed by doctors from King's College Hospital) at the *Churchill Clinic* (see page 94), where women can go without a GP's referral. There are plans to open other clinics elsewhere in the country.

HRT is available on the NHS. Your own GP may prescribe it for you, or he or she may refer you to a menopause clinic, or a hospital-based specialist. If your GP will not do this, or if you would rather have private treatment – at the Amarant Trust clinic, for example – expect to pay about £100 for the first year's treatment. Of course, once the dosage has been worked out, you could always go back to your GP and ask if he or she will now prescribe HRT on the NHS.

Alternative treatments

Although many women are enthusiastic about HRT, others are opposed to the idea of using hormones in this way, and prefer natural methods of coping with the symptoms of the menopause.

You could consult a herbalist or a homoeopath, and also check with your Community Health Council to see if there is a menopause self-help or support group locally.

If you are interested in self-help measures, there are two books you might find it useful to read – *Menopause, The Women's View* by Anne Dickson and Nikki Henriques, and *Overcoming the Menopause Naturally* by Caroline Shreeve.

MISCARRIAGE

Sadly, miscarriage is far more common than many women realise. It is estimated that between 15 and 20 per cent of all pregnancies miscarry, most of them during the first ten to twelve weeks. In fact, many 'late periods' are probably very early miscarriages.

I'm bleeding – am I going to lose the baby?

Any bleeding in pregnancy is worrying, but it does not mean you are definitely going to miscarry. So try not to panic (easier said than done, I know. I went into a blind panic when I had some spotting during my second pregnancy, but I went full term and had a healthy baby boy.) Many women have some spotting at the times when a period would have been due – it is a sign to take things easy around these dates.

You should contact your doctor, though, who will probably suggest you go to bed and stay there until a couple of days or so after the bleeding has stopped.

If you are also experiencing pain or cramps your GP may want to examine you to see if your cervix is opening, or he or she may refer you to hospital. You can, of course, go straight to your local accident and emergency unit. In hospital, ultrasound tests may be carried out to see if the fetal heart can be detected.

If the miscarriage is inevitable, some GPs will refer you at once to hospital where you may be advised to have a D and C (dilation and curettage).

If you miscarry at home alone, try to keep what has come away so that the doctor can examine it. Sometimes a miscarriage is incomplete and a D and C will be necessary to reduce the risk of infection and heavy bleeding.

How can I avoid a miscarriage?

Often the cause of an early miscarriage just cannot be pinpointed. Many doctors feel that miscarriage is nature's way of correcting mistakes, and that, upsetting though it is, in the long term it is probably for the best.

However, if you have several miscarriages in a row, you should talk to your doctor about preconceptual care and take extra rest right from the first days after possible conception. You could also ask about hormone injections, although different specialists disagree about their effectiveness.

If you repeatedly miscarry late in pregnancy, then ask your doctor about a referral to have some investigations carried out. It may be necessary to make sure your uterus and cervix are normal and functioning properly – you may, for instance, have a weak cervix, which can be treated by inserting a special stitch.

During your next pregnancy, you may be offered ultrasound scans and/or an amniocentesis.

Ectopic pregnancy

Sometimes the fertilised egg embeds itself outside the uterus, most commonly in the Fallopian tube – this is called an ectopic pregnancy. Usually the first symptoms are pain (often severe) and bleeding, but as these are the same kinds of symptoms that you get when you are having a miscarriage, an ectopic pregnancy can be difficult to diagnose. Some women also experience pain in their shoulders.

The danger is that if the tube ruptures, you can lose a great deal of blood very quickly, so if you have any reason to suspect you are suffering from an ectopic pregnancy rather than a miscarriage, do ask for an examination.

I speak from experience. When I started to bleed after a missed period, my GP said it was probably a miscarriage. Finally, after twenty-one days and two visits (on neither occasion was I examined), she suggested I went to the local casualty department. The doctor on duty was very off-hand, until he examined me, but then he could not get me to sign the operation consent forms fast enough.

If you have an ectopic pregnancy, it usually means you will have to have one of your Fallopian tubes removed. However, this does not mean you will never be able to have babies, or even that your chances are halved – I went on to have two with no problems.

Make the most of your enforced stay in hospital to ask the doctors all the questions you need answered.

Coping with the loss

Unfortunately, because miscarriage is so common, many doctors are fairly matter of fact about the whole thing, while for most women it comes as a shock. Coping with feelings of grief, anger or guilt, along with the body's hormonal upheaval, can be very difficult.

You might find it useful to contact the *Miscarriage Association*. If you send an s.a.e., you will be sent information about their publications and local support groups. (See page 95.)

POSTNATAL DEPRESSION

Women are usually warned to expect the 'baby blues' around three days after childbirth. As the hormone levels in the body drop, a few days of inexplicable weepiness are very common.

But the baby blues are very different from postnatal depression, which, in turn, is different from puerperal psychosis, an extreme, but rare, form of mental illness.

That said, there is no general agreement as to what exactly constitutes postnatal depression, although doctors these days are far more likely to be sympathetic to a woman suffering in one degree or another than they were in the past when you were likely to be told to 'pull yourself together'.

Some experts believe that postnatal depression can strike at any time in the first year after the baby's birth. Symptoms include extreme tiredness, feelings of futility, inexplicable sadness, anxiety, an inability to think straight, concentrate or remember things, loss of sexual desire and loss of appetite.

Many people think that PND is far more common than is usually acknowledged, and many women who suffer from it do not ask for, or get, the help they need.

Where to go for help

By the time you realise you have PND, your health visitor may have stopped visiting and your six-week check may be long past. However, you can contact your health visitor to ask her to come back and see you – you are her responsibility as much as the baby. Some health visitors run PND support groups.

You should also consider making an appointment to see your GP, who may be able to advise you about self-help measures, such as diet and vitamin supplements, or discuss treatment with hormones or anti-depressants. He or she may also know if the obstetrics/gynaecology department of any local hospital has anyone working on PND, so that you could be referred there for help.

You could also contact the *Association for Postnatal Illness*, enclosing an s.a.e. They will be able to advise you about treatment and support, and can help with referrals if you need medical treatment. (See page 93.)

Feeling you are not alone can make a big difference. The *National Childbirth Trust* runs postnatal support groups. You could contact them to see if there is one locally. (See page 96.)

A useful book to get hold of is *The New Mother Syndrome* by Carol Dix.

PREGNANCY AND CHILDBIRTH

For many healthy women, the nine months of pregnancy, culminating in the birth of their baby, give them their first real experience of specialists and hospitals. This can be a very happy and exciting time. But pregnancy also makes many women feel vulnerable, and the attitudes of the medical profession – from doctors to midwives – can make a great deal of difference.

Pregnancy is not an illness. Providing you are healthy and there are no complicating factors, there are a number of choices you can make about your care in pregnancy and during childbirth.

Planning pregnancy

Should I take advice on preconceptual care?

Experts agree that your lifestyle during pregnancy can affect your baby, but there is a growing body of opinion which holds that your lifestyle before conception can be important too.

Your GP may be able to offer preconception advice on the NHS, and some midwives and health visitors give informal counselling at their local clinics. Similarly, some of the larger hospitals run clinics along the lines of antenatal ones.

The *Spastics Society* produces a leaflet called *Healthy Mother, Healthy Baby*, and *Maternity Alliance* also has information on this subject. (See Useful Addresses; s.a.e.s please.)

Probably the best known of the voluntary organisations offering preconceptual advice is *Foresight*. They produce a number of booklets and will also put couples in touch with the nearest doctor running a Foresight clinic, so that they can be screened before they try to conceive. Consultation fees vary from clinic to clinic and from couple to couple, so telephone around to check prices before making an appointment.

Ideally, say the experts, you should allow at least three months, and preferably six, in which to make sure you are fit and healthy.

During this time you and your partner should eat a nutritious diet and cut down on consumption of tea and coffee (caffeine); avoid smoking or an excess of alcohol (some say *all* alcohol), as well as all drugs, including common ones like aspirin. (Of course, you should check with your doctor if you are on prescribed drugs.)

Experts also suggest that if you have been taking the contraceptive pill, you should switch to another form of contraception – such as the cap or condoms – for three to six months before trying for a pregnancy, in order to give your body time to return to normal.

Rubella

Even if you think you have had rubella (German measles) or were vaccinated against it, ask your doctor to check that you are immune before you get pregnant. This is important, because, although rubella is a mild illness, it can cause serious handicaps in babies if a mother contracts it during the first few months of pregnancy.

If it turns out you have no immunity, you should be vaccinated, but you should then wait three months before trying to conceive, as the vaccine itself is alive and might harm an unborn child.

Genetic counselling

If you are worried that you or your partner might have a

genetic condition or handicap that you could pass on to your children, ask your GP to refer you to a clinic where a counsellor can assess your case and explain what tests might be used during pregnancy if there is a risk. Most large hospitals offer this facility, and it is also available privately.

Pregnancy tests

You can buy DIY testing kits from a chemist. They all vary slightly in method and price, and can be used from one to five days after your period should have started. Ask the pharmacist for advice if you are unsure which one to buy.

Your GP may carry out pregnancy tests, or may send your urine sample to a lab for testing. You can also get a test done at family planning clinics (both NHS and private ones), at pregnancy advice centres and at chemists. In some cases there will be no charge for a test; elsewhere it may cost a few pounds. If the test is done there and then, you will get the results almost at once. If the sample is sent off to a lab, it could take a week or more.

All the tests involve a sample of urine: it is important for the sake of accurate results to take this from the first urine you pass in the morning, as this has the highest concentration of the hormone used to detect pregnancy. It will not be concentrated if you have been to the loo during the night, and you could dilute the sample if you have a cup of tea in bed before you head for the bathroom.

It is also important to collect and store the sample in a spotlessly clean bowl and bottle that have no traces of detergent. And it is no good keeping the sample too long. Same-day testing is crucial if you do not want to risk a false result.

Urine tests are generally 98 per cent accurate, but false results can sometimes occur because the urine was too diluted, contaminated, kept for too long, or because the test was done too soon.

Where to have the baby – hospital or home?

Childbirth expert Sheila Kitzinger suggests that even before you embark upon pregnancy, you should think about whether you would prefer to have your baby at home or in hospital.

For instance, if you decide you would like a home delivery, you may find that your own GP is not qualified to care for women in pregnancy and childbirth, or, even if your doctor is qualified, he or she is unwilling to attend a home birth.

In that case, you might wish to change doctors before becoming pregnant. The GPs who are so qualified are marked on the Family Practitioner Committee list of local doctors as obstetricians. The list is available at libraries, or you can get the information direct from your local Family Practitioner Committee or Community Health Council, whose addresses you will find in the telephone directory.

If you need to find another GP for a home delivery, you can register with one just for antenatal care, the delivery and postnatal care. You can stay with your own doctor for everything else.

There are all kinds of pros and cons to be weighed up when choosing where to have your baby. Only you will know what is important to you and your husband. *The Association for Improvements in the Maternity Services* produces some literature which may help you to make your decision. This includes the leaflets *Choosing a Home Birth* and *Choosing a Hospital Birth*. These both cost 50p. AIMS also publishes the *Directory of Maternity and Postnatal Care Organisations*, which is a guide to the various groups who offer advice and help in all aspects of pregnancy, childbirth and the first few weeks of life. This costs £1.00. You will need to add 30p for postage and packing for the first item, and 10p for any subsequent one. (See page 93.)

Many people feel that hospital is the safest place to give birth, although those who support the idea of home confinements challenge the statistics that are often claimed to prove this. However, in hospital there may be more kinds of pain relief on offer – epidurals, for instance – and, if there are any complications, medical skill and modern technology will be close at hand.

Sometimes there are medical reasons for going into hospital – if your baby is a persistent breech, or if you haemorrhaged with a previous labour, or if labour starts three weeks or more early, for instance.

Even so, despite the views of many consultants, many would argue that being a first-time mother (even a first-time mother over thirty) is not a good medical reason for a hospital birth.

Some women would much prefer to give birth in the familiar surroundings of home, where they can behave in the way they want to, rather than having to conform to whatever

66

the hospital rules and regulations are, and where the father will be an active partner rather than a barely tolerated bystander.

In theory, there are a number of options for mums-to-be. In practice, what is available depends not just on your own health and circumstances, but on local facilities and policies. Most babies are born in hospital these days, but even in hospital there may be alternatives.

Hospital births
Consultant units
Today, most babies are born in hospital and most are born in consultant units. In these you will be looked after by a team under the direction of a specialist. If there is more than one hospital in your area, you may be able to choose which one you go to. Once again, your own preferences will affect your choice. You might want somewhere like the maternity unit of a modern major teaching hospital, with all the latest technological equipment, or you might prefer a smaller local maternity hospital.

You can find out about different hospitals by talking to your GP and to your local health visitor. The local branch of the *National Childbirth Trust* (see page 96) will also be a good source of information, and you may find it helpful to get hold of a copy of Sheila Kitzinger's book *The Good Birth Guide*.

Most hospitals arrange tours round the labour and delivery wards, for women who are booked in. It may be possible to join one of these tours, or to go alone to look over the hospital before you decide whether to book in or not.

The *Pregnancy Book*, which is produced by the Health Education Council and should be available, free, to expectant mothers, gives a list of the kind of questions you might want to ask a hospital. These cover attitudes towards fathers being present during labour and delivery; whether or not women can move around in labour and give birth in any position they want; the hospital's policy on pain relief, induction, routine monitoring and other aspects of labour; whether or not there is a special care baby unit.

It also suggests asking about afterwards – are babies with their mothers all the time or is there a separate nursery? Will the hospital encourage and help you to feed on demand if that is what you want to do? What is the normal length of stay – and what are the visiting rules and hours?

It is also worth bearing in mind that two consultants in the same hospital may have different attitudes. When your GP refers you to a particular hospital, he or she will often refer you to someone he or she has worked with before. But you can choose your own consultant, provided you ask early enough. In practice, of course, it is unlikely that the consultant will actually deliver the baby. This is more likely to be done by the midwives, with a member of the consultant's team available if necessary.

GP units

In some areas there may be a GP unit, which will either be a separate unit, somewhere like a small cottage hospital, or part of the hospital's ordinary maternity wards. Here your baby can be delivered by your community midwife (or sometimes by a hospital midwife) and your GP. These units are generally used for low-risk births, such as second babies where delivery is likely to be normal.

The Domino scheme

Domino actually stands for domiciliary-in-out. What it means is that you are looked after for the most part by your local community midwife, who goes with you to hospital when you go into labour, and delivers the baby, perhaps with help from your GP or the hospital. Provided all goes well, she will take you home after, say, six hours and continue to look after you for the statutory ten days.

How long would I have to stay in hospital?

Different hospitals have different policies. In some areas you can ask if you can book an early discharge, in other words you may be allowed to leave either six or forty-eight hours after the birth, provided you and the baby are both well. If you do return home within ten days, your community midwife must, under the law, visit you for at least ten days after the birth to make sure everything is going all right.

Of course, you can discharge yourself from hospital at any time, providing you sign the forms. You would have to be very determined to do this against medical advice.

Home births

These days you may have to be persistent if you want a home birth, even if there are no medical reasons for you to have your baby in hospital. You may have great trouble in finding a

GP to provide care during labour and birth (see above), but, although it is illegal for an unqualified person to deliver a baby, except in an emergency, the law says you have the right to a home birth and that a doctor does not have to attend – a midwife is enough.

In fact, if your own doctor will not arrange for a midwife to attend you, then your District Health Authority has a legal obligation to do so. You should write (and keep a copy of the letter so that you have proof of your request) to the District Nursing Officer (Midwifery), or the Supervisor of Midwives for your local DHA. The address will be in the local library or the telephone directory, or you can ask your Community Health Council.

You should explain in the letter that you are expecting a baby on such and such a date and that you intend to have a home birth. Explain that your GP, Dr So and So of such and such address, feels/is unable to offer you medical care during your confinement and that you have been unable to find another doctor in your area who can.

You should then say that you would be obliged if the District Nursing Officer or the Supervisor of Midwives would make arrangements for a midwife to care for you during pregnancy and delivery at your own home, adding that you take full responsibility for your decision to have a home birth, and know that she will accept the responsibility of providing a competent midwife who will also have the facilities required to make your confinement as safe as possible.

It may be an idea for your partner to sign the letter also, and to send copies to the District Medical Officer, the chairman of the DHA and the chairman of your Community Health Council.

In some areas there are private midwives, operating independently outside the NHS. You might like to consider the possibility of paying for the services of one of these. To find out about local possibilities, contact the *Association of Radical Midwives*. (See page 93.)

Fighting to have a home birth can feel like a lonely battle, but you can get help and advice from *The Society to Support Home Confinements*. (See page 96.)

Private care

Even if you have private health insurance, it is unlikely that you will be covered for pregnancy and childbirth in general, although this may be possible if there have been problems in the past, or if problems actually occur.

In any event, it is best to check what cover you have before you commit yourself to anything. You may find you are only covered for antenatal care, but not the delivery.

If you do not have health insurance, or if your scheme does not cover you for pregnancy, you can still pay for private care yourself if you can afford it. Queen Charlotte's, probably Britain's best-known maternity hospital, in London, charges private patients a basic £226 a day just for accommodation. They estimate that the total bill (including fees for the obstetrician) could be around £2,500 for a first baby and £2,000 for subsequent ones, providing there are no problems. Outside London, the figure drops to somewhere between £1,200 and £1,800 for a straightforward labour and delivery.

In fact, there are a number of possible options which could determine the overall costs: you could have private antenatal care, but an NHS delivery; private antenatal care and delivery, both by a consultant; private antenatal care and delivery by a midwife at your home.

If you decide you want a consultant to deliver your baby, this could be in a private bed in an NHS hospital, or in a private nursing home, hospital or clinic. One thing to bear in mind when you choose is that if you *are* doing this on your insurance, you should make certain it covers everything and you should also check whether, if you have to be moved to another hospital for any reason, your current level of insurance would still be good enough. If there is any doubt, it might be worth asking the insurance company if you can increase your cover.

The advantages of private antenatal care are that you see the same person every time, you tend not to have to hang around to be seen (unless your consultant has been called out to do an emergency operation, for instance), and you get more time to ask questions and to talk things over.

Women who have had their babies in private hospitals and nursing homes say that they appreciated the privacy and the feeling that things were done for them rather than to them. One said: 'It was wonderful to have my own room rather than being in a large ward. I had a television and a 'phone and there were virtually no restrictions on visitors. And what was really nice was knowing that if you felt like a cup of tea at 3 a.m. when you were feeding the baby, you only had to ask for it.'

However, facilities do vary, as do hospital practices and consultants' preferences, and this is as true of the private sector as it is in the NHS. So even if you are planning to go privately, it is still necessary to do your homework before you make up your mind.

If it is the thought of ending up on a large ward full of other mothers and babies that worries you, you could find out whether your NHS hospital has any amenity beds. These are usually in smaller wards or single rooms, and may be available for a small daily charge if they are not needed on medical grounds for other patients. Having spent some time, post-natally, on a large Victorian-style ward after one baby, and in a small three-bedded room after another, I know that for me the small rooms win hands down every time. But other women may prefer the camaraderie of the larger wards.

Antenatal care

Throughout pregnancy, you will have regular check-ups to make sure everything is going well, both for you and the baby. Where you go and whom you see depends on where you are going to have your baby. By and large, if you are going to have the baby in hospital, then you will either go to the hospital antenatal clinic for all your appointments, or you will have what is called 'shared care' – this means you go to your own doctor for most of your check-ups, and in between you go to the hospital antenatal clinic.

If you are going to have your baby in a GP unit, under the Domino scheme, or at home, then you will probably go to your own doctor and midwife for all your antenatal care.

It is important to keep your antenatal appointments, even if you are working during pregnancy. *All women are entitled to paid time off for antenatal care during pregnancy: that is the law.* So do not let employers put pressure on you over this.

Although many hospitals have tried to improve the efficiency and friendliness of antenatal clinics, there can still be a lot of sitting about and waiting and the whole thing may seem very impersonal. Even if you are seeing your own doctor, you may feel guilty about taking up too much time by asking too many questions. You should not feel this.

If you do not know why something is being done, or what something means, ask. It often helps to write down a list of questions you want answered beforehand, and then take the list with you so that you will not forget anything.

71

If you are having your baby in hospital, you may only see the consultant at your first visit, and even then you may only be seen by one of the doctors working as part of his or her team. (If you want to see the consultant at any other time, ask the sister in charge of the antenatal unit.)

This first visit is probably the best time to discuss any particular wishes you have about the way you would like your labour and delivery to proceed.

You might want to talk about whether you are likely to be shaved or given an enema; whether your partner or a close friend will be able to stay with you all the time; whether your membranes will be ruptured, or labour accelerated in any other way; whether you can adopt any position you want, both for labour and delivery; how much choice and control you will have over various kinds and dosages of pain relief; whether you will be able to avoid an episiotomy; whether the baby will be delivered onto your tummy or taken away at once to be cleaned up.

Obviously, it is best not to be too aggressive, but it is no good giving in over everything you hold dear and then bitterly regretting it later. In 1984, a government report was published asking hospitals and medical staff to make labour and birth a more pleasant experience for women and to allow them the choices they want, providing these will not endanger the mother or the baby.

If the worst comes to the worst, you could remind the doctors of the report, but if, despite all your efforts, you still feel deeply unhappy, you might have to consider changing your doctor or hospital.

More hospitals will now accept the idea of individual birth plans, but whether you draw up something as formal as this, or whether you just end up agreeing certain points with the doctor, *make sure the choices you have made are written up on your records or your co-operation card*. That way, you have something down in black and white which may save arguments later.

Remember, too, that a plan is only a plan. And labour does not always go according to plan. In the event, some of the things you might have liked may not be possible.

The co-operation card

At your first antenatal visit, you will probably be given a co-operation card, which is used to record your health during the pregnancy. You should keep this card with you at all times, so that if you need medical attention, you have all the information needed.

The cards vary, but they all have one thing in common: they are not easy for the ordinary woman to make much sense of. Obviously, it can set your mind at rest, or help you to ask the right questions, if you know what the information on the card means.

Any column headed BP stands for blood pressure – what the doctor will be watching for is any significant rise in blood pressure during the last half of your pregnancy, which could be a sign of pre-eclampsia, a condition which can be dangerous for you or the baby.

The card will also probably give the length of pregnancy in weeks from the date of your last period, and there should also be a column for the height of the fundus, or the top of the womb. This is also a guide to the length of your pregnancy, so the two figures should be roughly the same. If there is more than a couple of weeks' difference, ask your doctor about it.

When you take in your urine sample, it will be tested: the presence of sugar can indicate diabetes; protein may indicate pre-eclampsia in later pregnancy; ketones are a sign that you may lack energy. The results of the tests will also be recorded on the card. A + sign, or **Tr**, means that a very small quantity of something has been found. **Nil**, a **tick**, or **NAD** all mean the same – nothing abnormal detected.

FH stands for fetal heart – **FHH** means fetal heart heard; **FHNH** means fetal heart not heard. There will also be a column recording which way up the baby is. After about thirty weeks, the baby usually settles lower, head down, ready to be born head first. **Ceph** or **Vx** are used to indicate this position.

Odema is another word for swelling, most often in the feet and hands. This is very common in pregnancy and is usually nothing to worry about. **Hb** stands for haemoglobin, and the levels of this are tested to make sure you are not anaemic.

If you do not understand something on the card, then ask. This is one of the few times in your life when you will have a chance to read some of your own medical notes – so make the most of it!

Special tests
Apart from routine checks on your weight, urine and blood pressure, you may be offered some other tests during pregnancy. These days more and more women are routinely

offered ultrasound, often referred to as a scan, at around sixteen weeks. High-frequency sound waves are used to build up a picture of what is happening inside your uterus. The sound waves are turned into a black and white picture on a small television screen. In some hospitals women are expected to have several scans, at others a scan is only used if there is a specific reason for needing the information it can provide. If you do not want a scan and do not know of any medical reason for having one, then you can refuse, but talk this over with a doctor before you make up your mind, so that you are fully informed.

It may be possible for your partner to be with you when the scan is done, and it has to be said that the first glimpse of the tiny form that is your baby can be a magical one. Do ask about this, but do not be too disappointed if the answer is no. Many hospitals and clinics (even some private ones) flatly refuse.

When the scan is being done and the picture appears on the monitor, it may not look like very much to the untrained eye. Do ask about it. You should get things explained to you.

Ultrasound can detect certain fetal abnormalities, but there are other tests – not carried out routinely – which also aim to do this. One is called chorionic villus sampling, but the more common test is amniocentesis.

This is usually done at about sixteen to eighteen weeks and may be offered to older women, who face a greater risk of having a baby with Down's syndrome, or in cases where there is known to be someone in the family with Down's syndrome, spina bifida, haemophilia or muscular dystrophy. Of course, you do not have to have the test: there is a small risk of miscarriage, or of damaging the baby. If the tests show that the baby will be born handicapped, then you will be offered a termination and you will then have to make a choice between that and bringing up a handicapped child.

It is vital that you know exactly why you are being offered an amniocentesis, or any other kind of test, and that you have all the information you need to make up your mind whether to go ahead with it or not. You should talk over the whole question with your doctor, the midwife or health visitor and your partner.

Antenatal classes
If you want to get the most out of the medical care available during labour and childbirth – whether you are having your

baby at home or in hospital – then antenatal classes are a good idea. The more you learn about the process of birth, the more you will be able to work with your body, and make the choices that will best help you to cope.

Most women start going to classes at around twenty-eight weeks, but you usually need to book up well before this. NHS classes are free and may be run by your GP, your local health centre, by local midwives or health visitors, or by staff at the hospital. Hospital classes usually include a tour round the wards, which can be helpful if you are having your baby there, as you can familiarise yourself with the surroundings and meet some of the staff you might encounter later.

The *National Childbirth Trust* has branches all over the country, and specially trained teachers run a variety of courses. The fees vary, depending on where you live, but as the NCT is a charity, it operates a fee-waiving scheme, so you will not have to pay if you really cannot afford it. In your area, there may also be yoga-based exercise classes, or classes run by local birth-centre teachers. Fees will vary. (See page 96.)

Prescriptions and dental care
While you are pregnant, and for a year after the baby is born, you are entitled to free prescriptions and free dental care. For free prescriptions, you need to fill in a form, which you can get from your GP, midwife or health visitor, and send this off to the Family Practitioner Committee.

For free dental treatment, just tell your dentist when you go. Now that dental charges have gone up, this is one 'perk' worth making the most of. Even the more expensive work – like capping teeth – will not cost you anything during this time.

Labour and delivery
No one can know in advance just what their labour will be like. These days – particularly if you are having your baby in hospital – there are various procedures which may be offered to you and it is worth thinking about these in advance, simply because when you are actually in labour, it is difficult to make calm, considered choices.

Of course, the reality may differ so much from the way you imagined things that you may change your mind on the day itself (I always said I wanted to avoid an episiotomy, if possible, but in the end I was only too glad when the midwife suggested one), but at least you will not be trying to take in a lot of new information between contractions. If someone suggests that an epidural might be helpful, or a midwife tells you she is going to rupture the membranes, you will know what is being talked about and can decide whether you want to argue the toss or not.

If you are attending NCT antenatal classes, the kind of techniques and procedures commonly used are bound to be discussed. Most books on pregnancy also give details. *The Complete Hand Book of Pregnancy*, edited by Wendy Rose-Neil, is a good example.

The kind of things you need to think about include:

Induction and acceleration of labour
There can be very good medical reasons for starting off labour artificially, but some doctors still routinely recommend induction if a woman is a week past her due date. However, some women (and some doctors) get their dates wrong and there can be as much risk to a baby born too early as to one born after forty weeks.

Different doctors also have different views about how long the average labour should be, and although, as with induction, there are times when there are sound medical reasons for speeding things up, you really need to know what the situation is in your own case.

You also need to consider the fact that whether you are given an oxytocin drip in your hand or arm (which, incidentally, often makes it hard to move about much), or have your membranes ruptured to start things off, you may suddenly find yourself faced with hard and powerful contractions, rather than building up more slowly to this stage. You are also very likely to be connected to an electronic fetal monitor.

Electronic fetal monitoring
Some hospitals use this kind of monitoring routinely; others only use a monitor if there is a particular reason. Some women like the idea and are reassured by it. Others do not like being wired up, because then they cannot move around as freely as they might wish. Once again, if this procedure is suggested, ask why it is being offered, as opposed to the more traditional way, where the midwife listens to the baby's heartbeat with a hearing trumpet.

In the past, some mothers have been told it is a question of staffing, and that there are not enough midwives available. But as someone will have to be there to check the machine anyway, this is debatable.

Pain relief
If you think you will want an epidural, this is something you should ask for early on in labour, as it takes time to set up and to take effect. It is the only kind of pain relief that gets rid of the pain altogether, but if you have an epidural, you will almost certainly have to be catheterised (as you will have no feeling in your bladder), you are likely to be more closely monitored and, statistically, you are more likely to have a forceps delivery with all the cutting and stitching this involves.

However, many women who have had epidurals argue that these are minor matters compared to the bliss of a painfree labour.

The biggest problem is that you cannot guarantee that you will get one just because you want one. Even in units where there is a resident anaesthetist on duty day and night, you will only get your epidural if he or she is not doing something else at the same time.

Pethidine is the most commonly used drug for pain relief, although it does not dispel pain in the same way that aspirin works on headaches. It actually dampens down the nervous system, thus helping you to relax and cope better. It takes about twenty minutes to take effect, and between two and four hours to wear off. The amounts given in each injection can vary from 50 to 200 mg, although the average dose today tends to be 75 or 100 mg.

If you are not sure you really need anything, you could always ask for a small dose, say 50 mg. And if you change your mind while it is being dispensed, you do not have to have it anyway – it can be sluiced away.

Always ask for an internal examination before accepting pethidine – you may be further along than you think. Using Entonox (gas and air) may be enough. Ask for this, if you want it, even if it has not been offered. (All home midwives carry it, too.)

Forceps
The rate of forceps deliveries varies from hospital to hospital, and, although there could be a number of explanations for this, it is possible that the attitudes of the doctors and

midwives play a significant part. You are often advised to have a forceps delivery if the second stage of labour is prolonged. The trouble is, different obstetricians have different ideas of how long too long is. Many have a definite time limit.

If you are anxious to avoid a forceps delivery, there are a number of things you could try. Sheila Kitzinger suggests you explore the effect of not pushing at all for several contractions. It may also help if you change position, getting into a more upright posture, by kneeling or squatting, so that you have gravity working with you rather than against you.

Midwives often ask partners to leave for a forceps delivery. If you cannot get permission for your partner to stay from the doctor who will be doing the delivery, it may be an idea for him to return as soon as he hears a baby cry. Everyone will be too busy to turn him out at that point, but, equally, they will also be too busy to call him back straightaway either.

Caesareans

About one in ten babies is now delivered by Caesarean section and the percentage of labours that end this way is rising all the time. Sometimes there is no other safe way to deliver a baby: perhaps the placenta is covering the cervix or is very close to it; perhaps there are signs that the baby is in distress or has stopped growing; perhaps it is clear that the baby's head is too large to go through the mother's pelvis; perhaps the baby is lying across the uterus, instead of head down.

Sometimes conditions like these can be diagnosed in advance, in other cases problems may only become apparent during labour. Either way, a Caesarean will be necessary. In other situations, however, the question of whether or not to carry out a Caesarean will be a matter of judgement and professional opinion, and different doctors may well take differing views.

For instance, some doctors feel that if, in a previous pregnancy, a woman had to have a Caesarean because her cervix did not dilate fully, she should automatically have a Caesarean the second time round too. Others think any sign of fetal distress, however minor, justifies emergency surgery. Some doctors believe all breech babies should be delivered by section. Others disagree.

You may be told at some point during your antenatal care that you will need a Caesarean, or an emergency Caesarean may be indicated during your labour and you will be asked to sign the consent form for the operation. You should try to make sure you are clear about the reasons why the doctor is recommending a Caesarean, and if you want to try to deliver vaginally, you should make your views known.

For instance, it is not a hard and fast rule that if you had to have a Caesarean first time round, you will have to have one the next time. If your consultant suggests this, ask about the possibility of a trial of labour. If your doctor seems to be working under a 'better safe than sorry' principle, or seems at all hesitant as to whether the operation is essential or not, you could ask for a second opinion.

If you do end up having a Caesarean, it is worth checking out the possibility of having it carried out with an epidural rather than a general anaesthetic, although this may not be possible in certain circumstances or in cases of real emergency. There are many advantages to having an epidural Caesarean – you will be awake when your baby is lifted out and should be able to hold and feed your baby within minutes; the chances are that you will feel better afterwards than if you had a general anaesthetic; your partner is more likely to be allowed to stay with you throughout.

Incidentally, although the practice of persuading women to have elective Caesareans to fit in with the doctor's personal commitments is rare in the NHS, it still happens sometimes in private practice. If you have got your dates wrong, or your baby is bigger than average for its dates, there is a slight danger here of delivering a baby prematurely.

Episiotomies
These days, episiotomy is used much more routinely than it used to be and many obstetricians argue that a cut is easier to repair than a tear. However, many women suffer a great deal in the weeks (and in some cases the months) after childbirth, from discomfort, pain and even infection as a result of an episiotomy, and some experts are convinced that a cut should only be made if there is a real risk of bad tearing, or if the baby is in distress and needs to be born quickly.

This is yet another of those areas which you really need to sort out with the midwives and hospital staff before you go into labour, but if you are faced with a choice at the last minute, you can, at least, ask why an episiotomy is being suggested.

It is also worth knowing that although midwives can cut, they are not allowed to stitch, so you may have to wait a while for a doctor to come and do the repair work. This also applies to midwives who deliver babies at home.

When can I say 'no' to something?

You cannot insist on delivering your baby in a certain way (whether you want to squat or have a Caesarean) although the Royal College of Obstetricians and Gynaecologists has said that women should be allowed to give birth in the way they wish, provided it is safe in their particular case.

However, you can refuse any treatment offered to you, unless it is an emergency. This could apply to pain-killing drugs or even induction if there appeared to be no good reasons for it.

Afterwards

When you are expecting a baby, it is very hard to think beyond labour and delivery. But giving birth is just a beginning, and when it sinks in that there is now a tiny baby to care for, even the most confident women may have pangs of doubt about their ability to cope.

Who is there to help?

While you are in hospital, there will be nurses and midwives who will show you how to do the basics, like changing nappies and bathing babies. Even if you went to parentcraft classes, there is a world of difference between practising on a doll and coping with a wriggling, screaming baby.

Hospital routines and practices vary. It is more common than it used to be to have babies roomed with their mothers day and night, rather than wheeled off to a nursery, but while you may be encouraged to have your baby in bed with you in one place, it may still be totally banned in another.

Even with the best will in the world, whatever system the nursing staff operate is bound to upset someone. With the current emphasis on breast feeding, some women are made to feel like pariahs if they choose to bottle feed from the start. However, if you want to do something differently, then you should ask.

Some women find it difficult to breast feed in hospital, despite the help that may be offered, but once back at home, in familiar surroundings and away from what may seem to be critical eyes, things often settle down.

Once you get home, you are likely to be visited by the

80

community midwife, who must come every day until ten days after the birth and may continue to come longer. At around this point, you will also be visited by your health visitor, who may be attached to your GP's surgery or to the local health centre. If you need help or advice between visits, contact your health visitor. That is what she is there for.

Some health visitors also run postnatal support groups, as does the National Childbirth Trust. The Trust also has breast-feeding counsellors and people who will give support to mothers with sick or premature babies. To find your local branch, ring the London headquarters. (See page 96.)

Under certain circumstances, you may qualify for a home help who will help with housework and shopping for an hour or so each day. Ask your health visitor about this if you feel you need this kind of support.

Some women feel that it is worth employing a maternity nurse for the first month or so. These are usually qualified nursery nurses whose job is to help you care for the baby. An alternative would be a temporary mother's help, to take over some of the housework. Both mother's helps and maternity nurses usually expect to live in, and they can be expensive. You can find this kind of help – and check out the prices – by contacting the private agencies who advertise in publications like *Lady* magazine. You can also advertise yourself.

Baby clinics

Baby clinics, run by the District Health Authorities, are often held at local health centres. Your GP, health visitor, or the Community Health Council will be able to give you addresses and times.

If your baby is ill, you should go to your GP, as only he or she will be able to prescribe medicines for specific illnesses, but there is usually a doctor at the clinic you can talk to if you are worried about something. There will certainly be health visitors you can see.

The clinic doctor will also carry out regular developmental checks and may give immunizations if these are not done by your GP.

Usually the baby clinic is where you go to have your baby weighed and where you can, if you wish, chat to the health visitor about all the everyday problems of sleeping, feeding, potty training and so on. It is also a place where you can meet other mothers.

Alternative Therapies

Remedies for minor ailments

As it is best to avoid taking drugs of any kind during pregnancy, coping with some of the minor ailments, which can be so common, can be difficult. However, alternative remedies are generally considered to be safe and you may find them helpful.

There are herbal and homoeopathic remedies for conditions such as morning sickness, heartburn and insomnia, but it would be wise to consult a qualified homoeopath or herbalist, rather than treating yourself with something bought over the counter. (For details on how to find a practitioner see page 91.)

Yoga exercises may also help if you suffer from backache, heartburn or constipation. To find a teacher near you, write to the *West London Birth Centre*, including an s.a.e. (See page 97.) Or check the list of adult education classes run by your local authority – even if a yoga teacher will not accept pregnant women, he or she may know of another teacher who will. Or you could contact the *Iyengar Yoga Trust*. (See page 95.)

Osteopathy can also be used for backache. *The British School of Osteopathy* runs a special pregnancy clinic in London, where you can have a series of osteopathic treatments to prepare for labour and delivery. (See page 94.)

Preparing for labour

Raspberry leaf tea is said to tone up the uterus ready for labour. Homoeopaths often recommend caulophyllum, which is said to promote quicker, more efficient labours.

Pain relief during labour

Acupuncture can sometimes be a very effective alternative to drug-based pain relief, but you would have to find a private acupuncturist willing to treat you and, if you were having the baby in hospital, you would have to get the consultant's permission for the acupuncturist to be present.

TENS, which stands for transcutaneous nerve stimulation, is another alternative, and may be available in your hospital. A hand-held box can be placed at certain points of the body, and the electrical impulses it gives off aim to block the pain messages to the brain and stimulate the body's own pain-relieving hormones, called endorphins.

The hospital physiotherapist, or the midwives, should know

82

if TENS machines are available (they are often used to relieve the pain felt after sports injuries). Ideally, you would need to experiment with a machine before you go into labour, so that you know how to use it.

After the birth
Alternative remedies are available for soreness and bruising – arnica is most commonly recommended. Herbalists and homoeopaths can also suggest remedies to help you breast feed, either by prescribing things which are supposed to increase your milk supply, or suggesting treatments to soothe sore nipples.

Yoga and meditation can help to relieve tension.

It may also be worth consulting a herbalist or a homoeopath if you suffer from postnatal depression.

PREMENSTRUAL SYNDROME (PMS)

These days, doctors tend to use the term premenstrual syndrome rather than premenstrual tension, because there can be a whole gamut of physical and medical symptoms associated with the approach of menstruation, other than a build up of tension. Not all GPs are sympathetic when it comes to PMS, but others take a great interest and can offer a good deal of help.

Before you go to your GP, it is a good idea to keep a menstrual diary, charting the various symptoms you get and the days of the month when they are present. If the symptoms appear only in the two weeks before a period, and disappear within forty-eight hours of starting to bleed, then PMS is indeed a probability.

Clinics
If you think you need help that your GP cannot, or will not, give, then you could try asking your local family planning clinic, although the range of services they can now afford to offer is diminishing. However, your own GP, or a family planning doctor, may be able to tell you whether there is a PMS clinic at any of your local hospitals. Well women clinics, if there are any near you, can also advise on PMS. You can ask about these at your local library, or by telephoning the

Community Health Council. Some Community Health Councils produce free leaflets on PMS.

The number of PMS clinics operating under the NHS is small. London is better served than elsewhere – there are clinics at UCH, the Royal Free, St Thomas's and the Elizabeth Garret Anderson hospitals, for instance – but even so, the waiting lists are long.

Self-help

Different clinics use different methods of treatment, and some you could try yourself. The use of evening primrose oil, vitamin B6 and a change in diet have helped some women.

The National Association for Premenstrual Syndrome can send you some factsheets and put you in touch with a local self-help group. The factsheets are free, but if you pay £6 for an annual membership, you also get a quarterly newsletter which will keep you up to date about research and other information.

Private care

As is often the case, you may find it easier to get treatment or help privately, rather than under the NHS.

For example *The Women's Nutritional Advisory Service* offers a six-month plan, by post, for tackling PMS, at a cost of £36. They also hold clinics in Brighton and London.

Women's Health Concern provides a specialist advisory service for PMS sufferers, and publishes a book and leaflets on the subject.

The Women's Therapy Centre runs support groups and holds workshops on PMS.

The *Family Planning Information Service* has a helpsheet on *Pre-Menstrual Tension*, which gives advice on how to chart your symptoms and provides some useful self-help tips on diet, exercise and alternative remedies. (See pages 93–97.)

SEX-RELATED PROBLEMS

These days you only have to pick up a paper or switch on the television to find yourself faced with some aspect of sex. Because sex is so widely discussed, it would be natural to assume that it does not pose any problems for women today.

Of course, this just is not the case. If anything, it is harder than ever now for women to admit to confusion, ignorance or doubts about their sexuality. Not only are there all the practical issues to worry about, from birth control (see Contraception) to sexually transmitted diseases (see Aids and Vaginal Infections), but there are all the emotional ones too.

There are still hundreds of women who do not enjoy their sex lives, who find it hard to reach orgasm, who experience a loss of libido. There are also those who find intercourse painful or impossible, and those whose partners experience premature ejaculation or secondary impotence.

Many couples still find it difficult to talk about sex, but unless you can discuss it honestly and openly (not when you are making love, but at another time when the stress and anxiety levels are not so high) any problems you are having will persist. A book you may find helpful is *Sexual Happiness* by Maurice Yaffe and Elizabeth Fenwick. Using questionnaires, charts and techniques based on established clinical procedures, it offers a self-help approach.

The Family Planning Information Service has a helpsheet called *Common Sexual Problems*, which outlines the most common difficulties and provides information on how to find out more. As it says, talking about what has gone wrong is often the first step. But if you really cannot talk through your problems – or if talking is not enough – then you should consider getting some outside help.

How to get help

Your GP should be able to give you reassurance and advice about sexual problems, and some GPs have even had special training in sexual therapy. However, many women feel uncomfortable talking to their family doctor about sex – and many GPs feel just as uncomfortable talking to their patients about sex.

It is also a fact that GPs often do not have the time available per patient to explore these kinds of problems as fully as they might wish. However, your GP should know where help is available.

Sometimes sexual difficulties are a symptom that all is not well in a relationship. Often counselling, rather than sex therapy as such, will be more appropriate. If you think this may be the case, then you can contact *Relate* (see page 96), through the national Marriage Guidance Council. (You do not have to be married.)

However, a couple may have a good relationship, but still be experiencing sexual problems. Under these circumstances, some kind of sexual therapy may be appropriate.

Sexual therapy has been available in Britain since the 1970s. A number of different centres have been set up under different auspices, and these are run by a variety of practitioners, such as psychologists, psychiatrists, doctors and counsellors. Some parts of the country are better served than others, and while some centres operate free under the NHS, others charge.

Some family planning clinics run sexual difficulty sessions, and all will offer commonsense advice; the Family Planning Information Service keeps up-to-date information. Relate trains its own therapists and tries to provide a national service. Clients are asked for a contribution and agree on an amount per session – the average is between £3 and £10 – but if you cannot afford to pay anything because you are unemployed, or on a very low income, you will not be turned away.

The *Institute of Psychosexual Medicine* (see page 95) and the *Association of Sexual and Marital Therapists* can also provide information about specially trained doctors or clinics in your area. If you want help on the NHS, you can always suggest that your GP contacts one or other of these so that a referral can be arranged.

Incidentally, many people worry that sexual therapy will mean having to perform in front of a therapist. This is not the case. In fact, many therapists begin by banning intercourse altogether (this takes away stress and anxiety) and any form of contact between the couple takes the form of tasks to be carried out at home.

For younger women, the *Brook Advisory Centres* offer counselling on emotional and sexual problems. The *Women's Therapy Centre* runs a number of workshops on topics such as sexuality for women, and women therapists offer counselling and psychotherapy.

SPOD, the *Association to Aid the Sexual and Personal Relationships of the Disabled*, can help with special problems if you or your partner are disabled. (See pages 93–97.)

SMOKING

These days, we are all aware that smoking is bad for us – and the smoking rates have been going down. However, all the evidence points to the fact that women have been giving up smoking more slowly than men.

In addition, one government survey has found that in secondary schools as many girls as boys smoke, and another report has shown that, between 1984 and 1986, the proportion of female smokers in their early twenties actually rose – from 36 to 38 per cent.

It has been argued that women find it harder to stop smoking than men, but a careful study of the available data suggests this is not the case. Nevertheless, as any woman who has tried to give up cigarettes knows, turning into a non-smoker can be difficult. So where can you go for help?

GPs

According to Ash (Action on Smoking and Health), it has been shown that with simple, but firm advice to stop smoking, plus a leaflet (the Health Education Authority produces one, *A Smoker's Guide to Giving Up*) and the warning of a follow-up check, family doctors can help about 5 per cent of their patients to stop smoking.

You could also ask your GP about Nicorette, a chewing gum which contains nicotine and aims to deal with nicotine withdrawal. This is not a magic substance which will help you quit with no effort at all, but some people find it helps in the early days. You need to be taught how to use it properly and safely, though, and you should have proper counselling and follow-up checks.

You can only get it on prescription, so you will have to see your GP if you are interested, but you will also have to pay for a *private* prescription as it is not one of the drugs available on the NHS.

Smoking-withdrawal clinics

Some people find it helpful to go to a smoking-withdrawal clinic. However, finding one locally may not be easy. You could ask your GP or your health education unit, which you will find listed under your local health authority in the telephone directory. Private operators or therapists may advertise in the classified columns of your local papers.

QUIT, the National Society of Non-Smokers runs intensive five-day courses. A small charge is made. (See page 96.)

DIY methods

The majority of people who stop smoking do it by themselves, but experts agree that the best way is to plan your campaign carefully. You can get advice from *Ash* by sending an A4 self-addressed envelope with a 20p stamp. (See page 93.)

QUIT (see above) also provides information and advice.

A book called *Kick It*, by Judy Perlmutter, gives details of a five-day stop-smoking programme based on techniques used at an American clinic. You may find this useful.

Alternative therapies

Hypnosis and acupuncture may help, but you need to be highly motivated. Neither technique can make someone give up if she does not really want to. To find a therapist, you could contact *The British Acupuncture Association* or *The British Hypnotherapy Association*. (See Useful Address.)

TRANQUILLISERS

When people talk about drug addiction, most of us assume they mean drugs like heroin or cocaine. In fact, many thousands of women become addicted to tranquillisers like Valium, Librium and Mogadon.

Often the addiction happens without the woman realising it. Only when she decides to stop – or her GP reduces the dosage or stops prescribing at all – do the withdrawal symptoms strike.

Coming off the pills

If you suspect you might be addicted to tranquillisers, you should talk to your GP about coming off the pills. Do not try to go 'cold turkey', that is, just stop completely. Your doctor will probably advise reducing the dosage gradually so that your body gets used to smaller and smaller doses in stages.

Your GP may be more than happy to help you through the withdrawal stage, but if your doctor is not sympathetic, or resents the implication that he or she does not know his or her job (after all, who prescribed the tranquillisers in the first place?) then you could contact a support group.

TRANX was set up by a former addict, Joan Jerome, in 1983. *Release* has leaflets on tranquillisers, and lists of self-help groups. You can also contact *MIND*. (See page 95.)

VAGINAL INFECTIONS AND SEXUALLY TRANSMITTED DISEASES

As most women are aware, the vagina produces natural secretions which keep it clean and healthy. The secretions may vary throughout the menstrual cycle (indeed, noting the variations is one way of using natural family planning methods), but variations which are out of the ordinary may be a warning signal of possible infection.

Rashes or sore spots on the genitals are also a sign that you should seek medical advice.

Not all infections are sexually transmitted – pregnant women and women on the pill are particularly susceptible to thrush, for instance – but some may have serious consequences if left untreated and this is why getting a correct diagnosis is important.

Where to go for help

You can go to your GP, but as lab tests will probably be necessary to establish the cause of the problem, it may be better to go direct to a Special Clinic. You can find out where the nearest one is by telephoning a family planning clinic, the out-patients department of a local hospital, or looking in the telephone directory under Venereal Diseases.

A visit to a clinic is not as embarrassing as many people fear it will be. The staff are generally friendly and non-judgemental. They will also observe confidentiality, and will not inform your GP of your visit, although, as always, it is in your own best interests that your doctor knows about any treatment you have had.

Self-help

As the old saying goes, prevention is better than cure, and there are a number of things you can do to prevent infection. You can practise safe sex – condoms do protect you from disease. You can be rigorous about hygiene.

If you are plagued by recurring bouts of thrush, you should not wear tight trousers, tights or nylon knickers, and you should not use powerful detergents to wash your underwear. Avoid soap when washing your vagina, do not use a flannel, and pat the vagina dry afterwards. Cut out sugar and only take antibiotics if your doctor insists.

Alternative therapies for the treatment of thrush include

bathing in salt water and putting *live*, plain yoghurt (obtained form health food shops) into your vagina, either by soaking a tampon or using a syringe.

Your local health education unit, if you have one, may have free leaflets or information packs, and *Women's Health Concern* produces two publications, *Sexually Transmitted Diseases* and *Feminine Hygiene*, and may be able to help you with any other information you need. There is also a relevant chapter in WHC founder, Joan Jenkins's book, *Caring for Women's Health*, available through the organisation. (See page 97.)

If you suffer from herpes you might like to contact the *Herpes Association* (see page 95), enclosing a large s.a.e. for further information. (See also AIDS; Cystitis; Gynaecological Problems.)

OTHER SOURCES OF HELP OR TREATMENT

Well women clinics

Despite all the emphasis today on preventative medicine, many of us look after our cars better than we do our bodies. We do not necessarily wait for a car to break down before we put it in for a routine service, but how often do we put ourselves in for a check-up?

Well women clinics have been set up to encourage us to do this. The kind of services offered by these clinics may include screening for breast or cervical cancer, checks on blood pressure, height and weight, and help and advice on diet, period problems, vaginal discharge, menopause and pre-conceptual care.

Unfortunately, there is no central register of well women clinics: some are run by GPs, others are based at health centres or hospitals. Most operate on an appointments system, but some have a walk-in service.

There are also a number of private clinics or screening services. At *Marie Stopes House* in London, for instance, women can have a Medicheck, which costs £60 for a forty-five-minute consultation (see page 94). BUPA also carries out well women screening at its twenty-one medical centres – the service costs £95, or £146 if there is an examination by, and consultation with, a doctor.

As you can see, if you go privately, these check-ups are not exactly cheap. However, all the clinics run under the auspices of the NHS are free. Your GP should know what is available locally, or you could ask your community health council.

If you go for a check-up at one of these clinics and anything seems to be amiss, you will not be treated there. The usual process is for you to be informed of the problem and a letter sent to your GP.

Alternative medicine

In recent years there has been an increased interest in alternative medicine – a broad term which encompasses all kinds of different therapies that may have little in common apart from the fact that they cannot be called orthodox medical treatments.

These therapies include herbalism, homoeopathy, aroma-therapy, osteopathy, chiropractic, acupuncture and acupress-ure, and hypnotherapy. Women may find homoeopathic or herbal remedies helpful if they suffer from period pains or premenstrual tension. Yoga can be beneficial during preg-nancy, as can osteopathy. In fact, the whole gamut of female problems and conditions may respond to one or more of these therapies.

How to find a therapist
Your own GP may use some form of alternative medicine, or may be able to refer you to a specialist. Some hospitals have set up acupuncture clinics, and homoeopathy, for instance, has always been available on the NHS. There are five homoeopathic hospitals, in London, Glasgow, Liverpool, Bristol and Tunbridge Wells, to which you could be referred. There are a few GPs who are also practising homoeopaths, and most homoeopaths work in the private sector. In fact, whatever form of alternative medicine interests you, it is likely that you will have to go outside the NHS to find what you are looking for.

Even so, it is a good idea to talk to your GP first: a *Which?* survey, carried out in 1986, found that nine out of ten patients who had tried some form of alternative medicine had not told their doctor because they thought that he or she would disapprove.

However, some GPs are very interested in alternative therapies and your doctor may be able to recommend someone known to him or her. In any case, your doctor should know if you are having some form of alternative treatment.

If your GP cannot help, ask your friends. Then choose a practitioner who is registered with one of the alternative professional organisations. Do not forget to ask about fees – a course of treatment can turn out to be very expensive.

The Institute for Complementary Medicine can supply lists of the names and addresses of local acupuncturists, homoeopathic doctors, medical herbalists, chiropracters and osteopaths. They publish a year book, which is available from libraries, and which will answer most of your questions. You can contact them for advice and information about treatment, but they will not actually recommend anyone. (See page 95.)

The British Acupuncture Association will send you a register with a list of clinics and practitioners (all in the private sector) and a year book explaining the treatments. Currently, this costs £1.50. (See page 93.)

The British Homoeopathic Association can supply a list of local practitioners and other information if you send an s.a.e. (See page 93.)

The British Holistic Medical Association does not act as a referral agency, but produces a number of self-help tapes and books. (See page 93.)

The General Council and Register of Osteopaths has a list of osteopaths, all of whom have had four years' training and are fully insured. (See page 95.)

USEFUL ADDRESSES AND TELEPHONE NUMBERS

Accept, 200 Seagrave Road, London SW6 1RQ, 01-381 2112

Alcohol Concern, 3 Grosvenor Crescent, London SW1X 7EE, 01-235 4182

Alcohol Recovery Project, 68 Newington Causeway, London SE1 6DF, 01-403 3369

Alcoholics Anonymous, General Service Office, PO Box 1, Stonebow House, Stonebow, York YO1 2NJ, 0904 644026

The Amarant Trust, 14 Lord North Street, London SW1P 3LD, 01-222 1220

Anorexic Aid, The Priory Centre, 11 Priory Road, High Wycombe, Bucks, 0494 21431

Ash, 5–11 Mortimer Street, London W1N 7RH, 01-637 9843

Association for Improvements in the Maternity Services, Ms S. Warshal, 40 Kingswood Avenue, London NW6

Association for Postnatal Illness, The Institute of Obstetrics and Gynaecology, Queen Charlotte's Hospital, Goldhurst Road, London W6

Association of Community Health Councils of England and Wales, 01-272 5459

Association of Radical Midwives, 8a The Drive, Wimbledon, London SW20 8TG, 01-504 2010

Association of Sexual and Marital Therapists, PO Box 62, Sheffield

Association to Aid the Sexual and Personal Relationships of the Disabled, 286 Camden Road, London N7 0BJ, 01-607 8851

The Back Pain Association, 31–33 Park Road, Teddington, Middlesex TW11 0AB, 01-977 5474

The Breast Care and Mastectomy Association, 26 Harrison Street, Kings Cross, London WC1 8JG, 01-837 0908

The British Acupuncture Association, 34 Aldermay Street, London SW1 4EV, 01-834 1012

The British Association of Cancer United Patients (Cancer Information Service), 121 Charterhouse Street, London EC1M 6AA, 01-608 1661

The British Holistic Medical Association, 179 Gloucester Place, London NW1 6DX, 01-262 5299

The British Homoeopathic Association, 27A Devonshire Street, London W1N 1RS, 01-935 2163

The British Hypnotherapy Association, 67 Upper Berkeley Street, London W1H 7DH, 01-723 4443

The British Nutrition Foundation, 15 Belgrave Square, London SW1X 8FS, 01-235 4904

The British Pregnancy Advisory Service, 056 42 3225

The British School of Osteopathy, 1–4 Suffolk Street, London SW1, 01-930 9254

Broadway Lodge, Old Mixon Road, Weston-Super-Mare, BS2 49NN, 0934 812319

Brook Advisory Centres, Central Office, 01-708 1234

Cancer Help Centre, Grove House, Cornwallis Grove, Clifton, Bristol BS8 4PG, 0270 743216

Cancer Information Service, 01-608 1661

CancerLink, 46A Pendonville Road, London N1 9HF, 01-833 2451

Churchill Clinic, 80 Lambeth Road, London SE1, 01-928 5633

The Endometriosis Society, 65 Holmdene Avenue, London SE24 9LD, 01-737 4764

Families Anonymous, 88 Caledonian Road, London N1, 01-731 8060

Family Planning Information Service, 27–35 Mortimer Street, London W1N 7RJ, 01-636 7866

Foresight, The Old Vicarage, Church Lane, Witley, Godalming, Surrey GU8 5PN, 0428 794500

Freephone Drug Problems – dial 0 for operator

General Council and Register of Osteopaths, 1–4 Suffolk Street, London SW1Y 4HG, 01-839 2060

General Medical Council, 44 Hallam Street, London W1, 01-580 7642

The Harley Street Medical Advisory Service, 01-935 0691

Health Education Council, 78 New Oxford Street, London WC1A 1AH, 01-637 1881

Herpes Association, c/o Spare Rib, 27 Clerkenwell Close, London EC1R 0AT

Institute for Complementary Medicine, 2a Portland Place, London W1N 3AF, 01-636 9543

Institute of Psychosexual Medicine, 01-580 0631

Iyengar Yoga Trust, 223A Randolph Avenue, London W9, 01-624 3080

Kilmartin, Angela, 01-249-8664

LIFE, 0926 21587

Marie Stopes House, 01-388 0662

Maternity Alliance, 59 Camden High Street, London NW1 7JL, 01-388 6337

The Medical Advisory Service, 01-994 9874 (eve only)

MIND, 22 Harley Street, London W1, 01-637 0741

The Miscarriage Association, 18 Stonybrook Close, West Brecon, Wakefield, West Yorkshire, 0924 85515

Narcotics Anonymous, PO Box 417, London SW10, 01-351 6794/01-341 6066

National Association for Premenstrual Syndrome, 25 Market Street, Guildford, Surrey, 0483 572 715

National Association for the Childless, The Birmingham Settlement, 318 Summer Lane, Birmingham B19 3RL, 021 359 4887

National Childbirth Trust (HQ), 01-221 3833

National Council for One Parent Families, 01-267 1361

Natural Family Planning Centre, Birmingham Maternity Hospital, Birmingham B15 2TG, 021 472 1377

Natural Family Planning Service, 1 Blythe Mews, Blythe Road, London W14 0NW, 01-371 1341

New Approaches to Cancer, Addington Park, Maidstone, Kent ME19 5BL, 0732 848336

Patients' Association, Room 33, 18 Charing Cross Road, London WC2H 0HR, 01-240 0671

The Pharmaceutical Society of Great Britain, 01-735 9141
Pregnancy Advisory Service, 01-637 8962

QUIT, The National Society of Non-Smokers, Latimer House, 40–48 Hanson Street, London W1P 7DE, 01-636 9103

Relate, The National Marriage Guidance Council, 0788 65675

Release, 1 Elgin Avenue, London W9, 01-289 1123 (emergency: 01-603 8654)

Society of Family Practitioner Committees, 0202 893000

Society to Support Home Confinements, 17 Laburnham Avenue, Durham DH1 4HA, 091 386 1325

Spastics Society, 12 Park Crescent, London W1N 4EQ, 01-636 5020

Standing Conference on Drug Abuse, 1 Hatton Place, Hatton Gardens, London EC1 8ND, 01-430 2341

Terence Higgins Trust, BM AIDS, London WC1N 3XX, Helpline: 01-833 2971

TRANX, 17 Peel Road, Harrow, Middlesex HA3 7DX, 01-427 2065

West London Birth Centre, 7 Waldemer Avenue, Ealing, London W13

The Wirral Hysterectomy Support Group, Rivendell, Warren Way, Lower Heswall, Wirral, Merseyside L60 9HJ

Women's Health Concern, Ground Floor, 17 Earls Terrace, London W8 6LP, 01-602 6669

Women's Health Information Centre, 52–54 Featherstone Street, London EC1, 01-251 6589/6530

Women's National Cancer Control Campaign, 1 South Audley Street, London W1Y 5DQ, 01-499 7532

Women's Nutritional Advisory Service, PO Box 268, Hove, East Sussex BN3 1RW, 0273 771366

Women's Therapy Centre, 6 Manor Gardens, London N7, 01-263 6209

FURTHER READING AND VIDEOS

Advice on Going into Hospital, Patients' Association
Beating Back Pain, Dr J. Tanner, Dorling Kindersley, 1987
The Bristol Programme, P. Brohn, Century Hutchinson, 1987
Can I Insist?, Patients' Association
Caring for Women's Health, J. Jenkins, Women's Health Concern, 1985
Choosing a Home Birth, Association for Improvements in the Maternity Services
Choosing a Hospital Birth, Association for Improvements in the Maternity Services
Common Sexual Problems, Family Planning Information Service
The Complete Hand Book of Pregnancy, ed W. Rose-Neil, Sphere, 1984
Directory of Independent Hospitals and Health Services, Longman, 1988
Directory of Maternity and Postnatal Care Organisations, Association for Improvements in the Maternity Services
Drug Problems; Where To Get Help, Standing Conference on Drug Abuse
Fat – Who needs it?, Health Education Council
Fibre in Your Food, Health Education Council
Feminine Hygiene, Women's Health Concern
The Good Birth Guide, Sheila Kitzinger, Fontana, 1979
Good Health Guide, Ealing Community Health Council
A Guide to Patients' Legal Rights, Patients' Association
Healthy Mother, Healthy Baby, Spastics Society
HIV Antibody: To test or not to test?, Terrence Higgins Trust
Hospitals and Health Services Year Book, Institute of Health Services Management
Infertility Tests and Treatment, Family Planning Information Service
Kick It, J. Perlmutter, Thorsons, 1986
Medical Directory, General Medical Council
Medical Register, General Medical Council
Menopause, The Women's View, A. Dickson and N. Henriques, Thorsons, 1987
The New Mother Syndrome, C. Dix, Unwin Paperbacks, 1987
Overcoming the Menopause Naturally, C. Shreeve, Arrow, 1986
A Patient's Guide to the National Health Service, Consumers' Association and Patients' Association, 1983

Planning a Pregnancy, Family Planning Information Service
Pregnancy Book, Health Education Council
Premenstrual Tension, Family Planning Information Service
Sexual Happiness, E. Fenwick and M. Yaffe, Dorling Kindersley, 1986
Sexually Transmitted Diseases, Women's Health Concern
A Smoker's Guide to Giving Up, Health Education Authority
Test in Time (video), Women's National Cancer Control Campaign
Understanding Cystitis, A complete self-help guide, A. Kilmartin, Arrow, 1986
Unplanned Pregnancy, Family Planning Information Service
Using the NHS, Patients' Association
Which? Way to Slim, Consumers' Association
Why Us?, A. Stanway, Thorsons, 1984
Woman's Guide to Health in Barnet, Barnet Community Health Council
A Woman in Your Own Right, A. Dickson, Quartet, 1982
Women and AIDS, Terrence Higgins Trust
Women and Alcohol, Alcohol Concern
Women on Hysterectomy, A. Dickson and N. Henriques, Thorsons, 1986

WHAT IS THE WI?

If you have enjoyed this book, the chances are that you would enjoy belonging to the largest women's organisation in the country – the Women's Institutes.

We are friendly, go-ahead, like-minded women, who derive enormous satisfaction from all the movement has to offer. This list is long – you can make new friends, have fun and companionship, visit new places, develop new skills, take part in community services, fight local campaigns, become a WI market producer, and play an active role in an organisation which has a national voice.

The WI is the only women's organisation in the country which owns an adult education establishment. At Denman College, you can take a course in anything from car maintenance to paper sculpture, from bookbinding to yoga, or *cordon bleu* cookery to fly-fishing.

All you need to do to join is write to us here at the National Federation of Women's Institutes, 39 Eccleston Street, London SW1W 9NT, or telephone 01-730 7212, and we will put you in touch with WIs in your immediate locality. We hope to hear from you.

INDEX

103

forceps delivery 77–8
Foresight 64
FPCs *see* Family Practitioner Committees
Freephone Drug Problems 49
further reading and videos 97–8

Gallagher, Mrs 15
General Council and Register of Osteopaths 92
General Medical Council 9, 15, 19, 22–3
genetic counselling 64–5
German measles (rubella) 64
Gillich rulings on contraception 43
Good Birth Guide (Kitzinger) 67
Good Health Guide (Ealing CHC) 10
GP(s) general practitioner(s) 14–20
  and abortion 26
  advertising and leaflets by 9–10
  and alternative therapies 91–2
  and breast screening tests 31–2
  and cancer 35
  can I insist on a woman? 16
  and cervical smear test 37
  changing 17–18
  closed lists 16–17
  and community nurses 20–1
  dealing with 1–4
  and drugs 48
  emergencies 18
  and family planning services 15, 41–3
  financial incentives to 14
  finding 14–16
  getting second opinion 19–20
  and gynaecological problems 51–2
  at health centres 16
  and hysterectomy 54
  and infertility 55–6
  making complaints 19
  and menopause 59–60
  and pregnancy and childbirth 64–9, 71, 75, 81
  private care 18–19
  referrals *see* referrals from GPs
  registering with 17
  relating pay of to performance 14
  services you have to pay for 19
  and sex-related problems 85–6
  shared care with hospital 15
  and smoking 87
  and tranquillisers 88
  units 68
  and well-women clinics 91
Guide to Patients' Legal Rights, A (Patients' Association) 11
Guy's Hospital 33

oxytocin drip 76

pain
  clinics 31
  relief during labour and delivery 77
Patients' Association, The 11
Patient's Guide to the National Health Service 11
pay of GPs, relating to performance 14
pelvic examination 52
pelvic inflammatory disease 52
periods, heavy painful or irregular 51–2, 53, 90, 91
Perlmutter, Judy 88
personal behaviour of doctor, complaints about 22–3
pessaries 41
pethidine 77
Pharmaceutical Society of Great Britain 47
pharmacists 47
physiotherapy for back pain 30, 82–3
pill, contraceptive 41, 42, 55, 64
Planning a Pregnancy (FPIS) 55
PMS (premenstrual syndrome) 3, 11, 53, 83–4, 91
  clinics 83–4
  private care 84
  self-help 84
PND *see* postnatal depression
post-coital service 44
postnatal care *see under* pregnancy and labour
postnatal depression (PND) 62–3, 83
practice nurses 21
preconceptual care 63–4, 90
pre-eclampsia 73
pregnancy and childbirth 63–83
  alcohol during 29
  alternative therapies 82–3, 91
    after the birth 83
    pain relief during labour 82–3
    preparing for labour 82
    remedies for minor ailments 82
  antenatal care 15, 71–2
    classes 74–5
  and community midwives 21
  co-operation card 72–3
  ectopic 61–2
  genetic counselling 64–5
  GPs qualified to deal with 15
  and health visitors 21
  home births 21, 68–9
  hospital births 67–8
    consultant units 67–8
    Domino scheme 21, 68, 71
    GP units 68
    length of stay 68

113